Rabies

THE FACTS

'It is even to be doubted whether any of the many diseases which afflict humanity, and are a source of dread, either because of their painfulness, their mortality, or the circumstances attending their advent and progress. can equal this (rabies) in the terror it inspires in the minds of those who are cognisant of its effects and who chance to be exposed to the risk of its attack, as well as the uniform fatality which terminates the distressing and hideous symptoms that characterise the disorder.'

GEORGE FLEMING
Rabies and hydrophobia: their history, nature, causes, symptoms, and prevention (1872)

Rabies

THE FACTS

EDITED BY
COLIN KAPLAN

OXFORD UNIVERSITY PRESS

1977

Oxford University Press, Walton Street, Oxford OX2 6DP

OXFORD LONDON GLASGOW NEW YORK
TORONTO MELBOURNE WELLINGTON CAPE TOWN
IBADAN NAIROBI DAR ES SALAAM LUSAKA ADDIS ABABA
KUALA LUMPUR SINGAPORE JAKARTA HONG KONG TOKYO
DELHI BOMBAY CALCUTTA MADRAS KARACHI

© Oxford University Press 1977

ISBN 0 19 264918 3

Set by Hope Services, Wantage
and printed in Great Britain by
Billing & Sons Ltd., Guildford and Worcester

Preface

With so many warnings being given about the dangers of rabies and the risk of its importation into Britain it seemed both sensible and timely to draw together in readable form essential information about the disease and the way it is spread. All the authors have either direct or indirect interests in the disease and its causative agent, and all have a very positive desire to keep it from our shores.

Nobody can doubt that the publicity campaign waged by the Ministry of Agriculture, Fisheries, and Food is necessary. We believe that in addition to such propaganda a sound background of fact about rabies can only help the efforts being made to keep it from re-entering Britain.

Chapter 1 discusses the epidemiology (or distribution) of rabies in Europe and other parts of the world, and shows how the disease is primarily one of animals, with infection of man being of virtually no significance in the further dissemination of the virus. It also describes the pathogenesis of the infection (i.e. the mechanisms of which the virus spreads in the infected host and causes the symptoms of the disease) and its relationship to transmission of the virus. Studies of the European epizooty show clearly that the red fox is by far the most important animal involved. Except in some special circumstances in the Americas and the eastern part of Iran, dogs (and cats) are much the most probable source of infection for man.

Brown and Crick (Chapter 2) describe the causative virus of rabies and discuss its relationship with a group of rabies-related viruses which have been isolated in various parts of Africa. In their studies Brown and Crick have been able to relate several biological functions of the virus to structural features, and have shown that a surface component (the glycoprotein) can be used to induce immunity to infection in animals even when it is removed from the virus and purified. This clearly has important implications for vaccine technology.

Chapters 3 and 4 by Warrell and Haig contain clinical descriptions of the disease in man and the more important of his domesticated animals. Warrell (Chapter 3) relates the symptoms of the disease in man to the involvement of the nervous system briefly described in Chapter 1. Haig (Chapter 4) emphasizes that abnormal behaviour is an important indication of the early stages of disease in animals and points out that awareness of this fact makes for early recognition of the disease in pets.

Macdonald and Lloyd (Chapters 5 and 6) consider complementary aspects of fox ecology and behaviour in Britain. It is generally agreed that if rabies is introduced into Britain it will probably be via a dog or cat brought in illegally while incubating the disease. It is likely that such an importation will be followed by an outbreak in pet animals if the imported case is not recognized in time; but spread to foxes can by no means be excluded. An understanding of the ecology and behaviour of foxes is essential if the occurrence of cases in wildlife is to be prevented from developing into a widespread epizooty. From their different starting points both Lloyd and Macdonald accept this, but both deplore any idea of wholesale slaughter of foxes before the event, and are doubtful of its efficacy should rabies become established in Britain.

Turner (Chapter 7) describes the vaccines which are available for the treatment of persons bitten by a known or suspected rabid animal. Although there have in the last few years been considerable improvements in rabies vaccines it is unlikely that the vaccines which are safest and most effective will be widely available in those countries with the greatest annual incidence of rabies. The newest vaccines are very expensive to prepare and are likely to be beyond the means of developing countries, where the greatest incidences of rabies are found. There are, nevertheless, potent and much improved vaccines prepared from animal brains which are relatively inexpensive to make.

The picture which emerges is of a serious, but not overwhelming, problem which is being attacked from many sides in a reasonably co-ordinated way by scientists using up-to-date concepts and research techniques. While rabies can never be eradicated world-wide, protection against it can now be widely offered — to animals as well as men — but it is still worth making considerable efforts to prevent its entry to those countries and regions lucky enough not to harbour it.

I should like to thank May & Baker Ltd for their help in providing photographs of rabid animals from the film *La Rage – Son Nouveau Visage*, and my wife for the trouble she took over the preparation of the index.

Reading   *Colin Kaplan*
November 1976

Contents

List of contributors

COLIN KAPLAN, M.Sc., M.B., Ch.B., Dip. Bact., F.I.Biol., F.R.C.Path., Professor of Microbiology, University of Reading.

F. BROWN, B.Sc., M.Sc., Ph.D., Head of Biochemistry Department, Animal Virus Research Institute, Pirbright, Surrey.

JOAN CRICK, M.Sc., Biochemistry Department, Animal Virus Research Institute, Pirbright, Surrey.

DAVID A. WARRELL, M.A., D.M., M.R.C.P., Consultant Physician, Clinical Lecturer in Tropical Medicine, Radcliffe Infirmary, Oxford.

D.H. HAIG, O.B.E., B.V.Sc., D.V.Sc., M.R.C.V.S., Head of Department of Microbiology, Institute for Research on Animal Diseases, Compton, Nr Newbury, Berks.

DAVID W. MACDONALD, B.A., Animal Behaviour Research Group, University of Oxford.

H.G. LLOYD, M.Sc., Pest Infestation Control Laboratory, Ministry of Agriculture, Fisheries and Food, Llandrindod Wells, Powys.

G.S. TURNER, B.Sc., Ph.D., Lister Institute of Preventive Medicine, Elstree, Herts.

1

The world problem

COLIN KAPLAN

Rabies has been and is still regarded in all parts of the world as one of
the most terrifying diseases known to man, and certainly as the disease
causing the most terrible death. It has, however, never occurred in mass-
epidemic form as the Black Death did and influenza still does. The
Black Death, caused by the plague bacillus carried by rats and spread by
their fleas, is estimated to have killed between a quarter and a third of
the population of Europe (including Britain) in the fourteenth century.
Influenza is estimated to have killed about 20 000 000 in the pandemic
after the First World War. Even in areas where the disease is prevalent
and virtually uncontrolled, deaths from rabies are not counted in
such numbers. In Sri Lanka, for example there are, on average, about
200 human deaths a year in a population of 12 500 000. The figure
for India is not known, but various estimates have been made; none
pretends to accuracy and almost all, in my opinion, are too low. At a
Seminar on Veterinary Public Health held in New Delhi a few years
ago by the World Health Organization, one of the participants, Dr C.W.
Schwabe, suggested that the annual number of human deaths from
rabies in India was 15 000. Although this is 50 per cent more than the
number obtained by extrapolating the Sri Lanka annual average to a
population the size of India's, I believe it is still too low. Nevertheless,
if the number of people dying of rabies each year in India were to be
twice as great as Schwabe's estimate, it would be very small beer,
epidemiologically, in relation to the annual mortality attributable to
gastro-intestinal infections. If, however, the disease is considered not as
an element in a statistical comparison but in terms of human suffering,
it is far more than can be contemplated with equanimity.

All warm-blooded animals are susceptible to rabies; but, according
to the World Health Organization's Expert Committee on the disease,
not all animals are equally susceptible. The most highly susceptible are
foxes, coyotes, jackals and wolves, kangaroo rats, cotton rats, and
common field voles. The group next most susceptible contains many
species which are important in maintaining reservoirs of infection in
wild life in many different parts of the world. Dogs are listed as only
moderately susceptible; but dogs are without any doubt the animals

1

most likely to spread the infection to human beings. In man, one of the manifestations of the infection – an inability to swallow liquids – has given the disease the name hydrophobia. Since the development of symptoms in man is sufficiently different from that in other animals, hydrophobia is a term used only to describe the disease in human beings.

Development of the infection

The cause of the disease is a specific virus (described in Chapter 2) which is spread in the saliva of infected animals. Probably the commonest method of transferring the virus in saliva is by the bite of a diseased animal. The virus is thus deposited in the tissues of the new victim and can start its cycle of infection and multiplication.

When Pasteur's colleague Dr Emile Roux first isolated and worked with the causative agent of rabies in 1881 he claimed that it travelled from the entry wound to the central nervous system via the nerves. This view was later challenged by others, and for many years – indeed, until quite recently – the way the virus spread in the infected host from entry site to the brain where it exerts its disease-producing effects, was disputed. There was much evidence in favour of the neural route, but its final acceptance was delayed. Sir Macfarlane Burnet, a truly great biologist, famous for his research in virology and immunology, wrote in 1955 about the general proposal that viruses which infect the central nervous system move in the peripheral nerves. He found it 'quite impossible to review the literature without accepting the existence of such movement and almost equally impossible to believe in its physical reality'. Today, largely because of the experimental work of Dr L.G. Schneider of the Federal Institute for Animal Virus Diseases at Tübingen in West Germany, Dr R.T. Johnson of Johns Hopkins University, and Dr G.M. Baer of the United States Center for Disease Control, it is generally accepted that, after its deposition in the tissues, the virus enters a peripheral nerve and moves steadily up the axon cylinder (the central part of the nerve fibre which carries the impulses or messages from the nerve cell) towards the spinal cord and thence to the brain. Since the days of Sir Macfarlane's qualified disbelief electron micrographs have been published which show, quite unequivocally, the presence of virus particles inside the axon cylinder. Not only rabies virus, but also others such as herpes virus have been demonstrated within the axon cylinder.

Once in the brain the virus multiplies in nerve cells in all parts of the organ. Infection of the cells of the limbic system which is closely associated with emotional behaviour is especially important. R.T. Johnson pointed out that this is the adaptation which, almost more than any other, is likely to drive the infected animal into frenzies of rage and so cause it to attack, and bite – and transfer the infection.

Having multiplied in the brain cells the virus then moves outwards to the periphery once more, still via the nerves. This time all the efferent or outgoing nerves are involved: not those of the voluntary nervous system only, but also those of the involuntary or autonomic nervous system. The virus is thus conveyed to practically every tissue and organ in the body including, of course, the salivary glands, and so finds its way into the saliva. The animal, driven to a pathological rage by the virus multiplying in the cells of the limbic system, makes unprovoked attacks and so infects new hosts and sets the whole process going once more. An infected animal in a quiet phase of the disease, or one suffering from the paralytic form of the disease, may contaminate a scratch or other small wound on its owner's hand by licking it. The important factor in spreading the disease is thus the transfer of infected saliva, and not necessarily the bite inflicted by the rabid animal.

Diagnosis

Until recently the diagnosis of rabies during life was a clinical one, depending upon the skill and knowledge of the physician or veterinary surgeon. After death the diagnosis could be confirmed by microscopical examination of the brain. The general appearance of the brain in rabies is not greatly different from its appearance in other inflammations (or encephalitides) caused by viruses. In 1903 Dr A. Negri of the University of Padua described some inclusions in nerve cells (neurones) of rabid brains which still bear his name. Negri bodies, when found, are specific indicators of infection by rabies virus; but cases occur in which they are very few or even not found at all. To overcome this difficulty, a usual part of the diagnostic process is a biological test: an extract of brain tissue of the suspected case is injected into the brains of laboratory mice.

The presence of Negri bodies in the brains of test mice is generally regarded as adequate evidence of infection by rabies virus, but there should always be a confirmation of any positive biological test, and confirmation can be made biologically by doing a neutralization test. This is done by mixing some of the extract of brain tissue with authentic rabies antiserum and inoculating mice with the mixture, while another group of mice is given extract without antiserum. If the mice of the first group do not die (though the others do) they have been protected by the antibody in the serum neutralizing the infectivity of the agent in the extract, which must therefore have been rabies virus.

When rabies virus is present, unprotected mice generally die in 7 to 14 days after the injection, but if the material being investigated is, for example, from a dog which has bitten somebody, or even several people, fourteen days is a long time to wait for a definite answer.

About twenty years ago a serological technique known as immuno-fluorescent microscopy was adapted to the diagnosis of rabies. The serological reactions, including neutralization and immunofluorescence, depend on what is called immunological specificity. A substance which stimulates the production of antibody by an animal is known as an antigen. Antigens combine specifically with the antibodies they evoke and there are various ways of demonstrating the combination. The property of immunological specificity is the basis for many different kinds of serological tests, i.e., tests made with serum as an essential component. In virology several serological tests are commonly used, of which the most important are neutralization, immunofluorescence, immunoprecipitation, and complement fixation which is a complex indirect test widely used in diagnostic laboratories. Most microbiological agents, including viruses, possess more than one antigen, but for purposes of identification of viruses there is usually one of overriding importance. In their discussion of rabies and rabies-related viruses in Chapter 2, Brown & Crick mention the 'spike' antigen which determines type specificity and the nucleoprotein antigen which is responsible for the rather wider group specificity.

Serological tests require the use of antisera specific to the particular antigens being tested for. These are generally prepared by inoculating rabbits with the relevant antigen, although other animals are sometimes used. For antiserum to an agent which is able to infect and perhaps kill the animal a non-infectious preparation is used. For rabies antiserum it is usual to immunize the animal with a vaccine-like preparation (see Chapter 7). The resulting antiserum may be regarded as a solution of antibody, or the antibodies (a particular species of protein in the serum) may be extracted from the serum and dissolved for use in a suitable solvent.

The basis of the immunofluorescent method is straightforward. A solution of purified antibody is labelled with fluorescein isothiocyanate or some other suitable dye. The labelled antibody is then reacted with a preparation of (or containing) the antigen which stimulated the production of the antibody in the first place. The antibody and antigen combine specifically. When the antibody-plus-antigen combination is examined with a microscope in light of appropriate wavelength (an ultraviolet lamp is usually used) the label attached to the antibody fluoresces brightly, indicating the presence in the preparation of the particular antigen being tested for. Since the method was originally used for diagnosis of rabies various improvements have been made in the sensitivity and specificity, and rabies virus antigens can now be recognized in infected cells with considerable certainty. Two further adaptations have made it possible to use immunofluorescent microscopy to confirm the diagnosis of rabies in living subjects. Both depend on the fact that the peripheral movement of virus from the central nervous system carries the virus to all parts of the body. In the first

4

method a clean glass slide is pressed against the cornea (the transparent part of the eyeball overlying the iris and pupil). Some of the corneal cells are deposited on the glass in an 'impression smear', which is examined by immunofluorescence. Because corneal impression smears do not always have enough cells the second method was introduced. This consists of taking a small piece of skin from the suspected case of rabies, freezing it to permit the cutting of very thin slices, and then examining these slices (or frozen sections) by immunofluorescence to identify virus antigen.

Especially in developing countries where rabies is a problem, not every pathology laboratory has a fluorescence microscope, which is expensive to buy and to maintain. An alternative method is now beginning to be used for labelling antibody. This depends on the use of certain enzymes and, in extensive tests, seems to be at least as sensitive as labelling with fluorescein, but has the advantage that expensive special microscopes are not needed for the recognition of the labelled antibody in the microscopical preparation.

The outcome of infection

The time between the deposition of the virus in the tissues and the onset of symptoms is the incubation period of the disease. As a rule, the further the entry site is from the head the longer is the incubation period. This is discussed by Warrell in Chapter 3 and Haig in Chapter 4 in relation to the disease in man and in animals. Every deposition of virus is not inevitably followed by disease. Experimental work in animals has shown clearly that some infections may be abortive and some of these may be followed by immunity. Abortive infection is not confined to rabies; it happens with many infectious agents. It is common with poliomyelitis virus when it is known as 'sub-clinical' infection, which also leads to immunity.

It is widely believed that the development of symptoms of rabies is a prelude to inevitable death, but this is a view which is increasingly being questioned. There is now acceptable evidence that at least in some animals recovery from rabies may not be an exceptionally rare event. In man, however, survival – or at any rate, well-documented survival – is so infrequent as to be regarded by many physicians with caution amounting to disbelief. The medical literature contains reports of two cases which seem to me to be acceptable. The first is that of Matthew Winkler who, when he was six, was bitten on the thumb by a rabid Big Brown bat (*Eptesicus fuscus*) in Lima, Ohio, USA. The second is that of a woman of forty-five in Argentina who was badly bitten about the left arm by a dog which died four days later with a clinical diagnosis of rabies. No post-mortem examination was made of the dog and no attempt was made to isolate rabies virus from it.

Treatment with suckling mouse brain vaccine (see Chapter 7) was begun six days after the dog died. Twenty-one days after the bite, before the course of vaccine had been completed, the patient developed mild symptoms which increased to severe involvement of the nervous system. She was treated vigorously but her eventual (although incomplete) recovery took more than a year. Rabies virus was neither isolated from nor demonstrated in either of these patients. Warrell inclines to the view that post-vaccinal accidents cannot be excluded in either case, and is not convinced that either had rabies.

Experimentally it has been shown in a variety of animals that antibody to rabies virus is never found in the cerebrospinal fluid except after infection of the nervous system with the virus. There is no reason to believe that human beings react any differently. Antibody to rabies virus has never been found in the cerebrospinal fluids of normal people immunized with potent vaccine; both Matthew and the Argentinian patient had considerable concentrations of antibody in cerebrospinal fluid and extremely high concentrations in the blood. The Argentinian patient's daughter, who was also bitten by the dog, was given a course of vaccine; her blood antibody concentration was modest compared with that of her mother, and there was no antibody in her cerebrospinal fluid. On balance, laboratory workers with rabies virus are inclined to accept that both these patients did, indeed, have rabies.

Epidemiology

The study of the causes and distribution of diseases is called *epidemiology*. Epidemiology was once strictly associated with its Greek roots, but usage has altered and it deals now not only with what is 'upon the people' but includes the study of the determinants of diseases occurring in all species. I use *epizootiology* in discussing in a particular sense the diseases of animals, and *epidemiology* when discussing the distribution of disease in a more general way.

Like other communicable diseases rabies appears in cyclical outbreaks, although this must, to some extent, be guessed from early literature. The keeping of more or less reliable statistics of disease began to be widely practised only in the nineteenth century. However, when there is general reference to madness in dogs and other animals by writers in many parts of Europe it is probably safe to assume that rabies was meant, and that a cyclical wave of infection was active at the time. There are statements by early authors which suggest that rabies was prevalent in the Middle Ages, not only in Europe generally but also in Britain. From about 1500 onwards rabies was widespread and frequent, largely among dogs but with many references to madness among wild beasts of many kinds. Foxes, badgers, and even bears were involved in epizooties (animal epidemics), but without doubt wolves were the most feared of rabid wild animals, since it was well appreciated that people savaged by rabid wolves were at much greater risk of hydrophobia than those bitten by mad dogs.

Another major European outbreak began early in the eighteenth century when the disease spread from Eastern European countries, involving both dogs and wild life. There was an increased prevalence of rabies in Britain from about 1735, and the number of infected animals seems to have increased during the next twenty to twenty-five years. London was heavily affected. Also, in the mid-eighteenth century, rabies was prevalent in the North American colonies; a high frequency of occurrences was reported in Boston and other towns. Significantly, further reports of rabies in and around Boston in 1770 and 1771 implicated not only dogs but also foxes, and the disease was regarded as a new one; but this is difficult to accept today. By 1785 the disease was active in all the northern states of the recently established United States of America.

The period of the Napoleonic wars and the twenty or so years after them coincided with another European outbreak of rabies. At the end of December 1803 foxes were seriously involved in the evolution of the epizooty. Many foxes were infected in the Jura region. Foxes were found dead 'and people, dogs, pigs, and other animals were bitten'. The epizooty continued until 1835, by when it had spread over the whole of Switzerland. The disease spread also into Southern Germany and invaded Württemberg, Baden, and Bavaria by 1820, and the Black Forest by 1825. It was present in Upper Hesse by 1824 and somewhat later reached Lower Hesse and Hanover. This serious epizooty of rabies in foxes continued until 1835 or later and the area affected was very much that which subsequently bore the brunt of the fox rabies epizooty of the 1960s. A notable difference between that earlier epizooty and the more recent one is that the foxes then were extraordinarily aggressive. 'They attacked people in the woods or on the public highways, even entering villages and during the continuance of the outbreak every kind of domestic animal suffered from the transmission of the virus by wounds occasioned by these creatures; even fowls were not exempt.'

Rabies continued to be widespread in Britain. Various parts of the country were alarmed from time to time, but the outbreaks were largely local, and such reaction as there was was also local. In 1864, however, the number of rabid dogs in the country increased greatly, especially in Lancashire; in June at least 1000 dogs were destroyed in Liverpool alone. By the next year the disease was more widespread in England: the number of human deaths from hydrophobia increased from twelve to nineteen. In 1866 the situation was clearly very serious; there were thirty-six deaths from hydrophobia, eleven of them in

Colin Kaplan

London and thirteen in Lancashire. The Metropolitan Streets Act was passed by Parliament in 1867 which empowered the police in London to 'seize all vagrant dogs'. The Act was put into force in June 1868 and the number of cases of hydrophobia was immediately diminished. The rest of the country was not so fortunate. The North of England continued to be plagued by the disease. It was widespread in Lancashire in the early Spring of 1869 with several human deaths and was reported in Yorkshire by the Autumn. From Lancashire it had spread not only to Yorkshire but also to the more northern counties, and thence both to Scotland and southwards. To indicate the way the disease travelled Fleming wrote in 1872 'A rabid retriever dog attacked and wounded several persons and dogs in and about Derby, Nottingham and Loughborough, in November. It was supposed the animal had been bitten in the commencement of the month near Wigan'. If the dog did, indeed, come from Wigan it had not only crossed the Pennines (presumably after the effects of the virus began to be apparent, two weeks or more after the infecting bite) but had covered a minimum distance of 100 miles, assuming it had moved only by the shortest routes between points on its itinerary. This is a good example, therefore, of the sort of distances a rabid dog could cover, and demonstrates the small chance there was of finding and stopping it, even at a time when a far larger proportion of the population lived and worked in the country than today. The local newspapers, the veterinary journals, and the *British Medical Journal* all carried frequent reports of the appearance of mad dogs and the death and disaster which followed their passage.

Huddersfield Justices of the Peace, either wiser than many or better-advised, issued proclamations that all dogs in the Borough be 'confined on suspicion of canine madness . . . every person who . . . suffers any dog to be at large, incurs a penalty of any sum not exceeding forty shillings, or . . . may be imprisoned for a period not exceeding fourteen days. All dogs found in the streets or highways will be considered to be at large unless held in check by a string, chain, strap or other fastening'. An effective method of controlling and preventing the spread of rabies was clearly understood, but only where its application was backed by the power of Parliament, as in the Metropolitan Streets Act of 1867, was the regulation of dogs successful in halting the epizootic spread of the disease and consequent hydrophobia in the human population. Yet, even in the absence of laws and local proclamations, there were people sufficiently knowledgeable and responsible to confine and destroy their own animals, not only when they developed signs of rabies, but even when there was suspicion that they might have been infected.

This is particularly notable in the history of some of the well-known fox-hound packs. In 1871 several hunting kennels reported the presence

8

of rabies. The Quorn lost the whole of the entry for that year, while the Albrighton Hunt, which had seemed in May to have had only a few young hounds of the year's entry affected, ended by destroying the survivors of the pack in November because new cases went on occurring. The Albrighton Hunt thus lost its whole pack of 29 couples. The Durham County hounds were also unlucky. 'The pack of 41 couples commenced the season under the most promising auspices, with a country well-stocked with foxes and every prospect of success . . .' The huntsman observed one of the new hounds behaving strangely, suspected rabies, and isolated the animal. The full symptoms developed and the animal died. 'Four hounds he had previously bitten were at once put down.' After a short lull other hounds developed unmistakable rabies. As soon as the symptoms appeared hounds were destroyed since it was clear none would recover. The subscribers to the hunt were consulted about 'the proper course to be adopted . . .' Should the pack be destroyed or an attempt be made to control the disease by isolating each hound? '. . . the meeting came to a unanimous resolution: "That it was a duty they owed to the country to sacrifice the whole of their gallant pack and to appeal to masters of hounds for a few hounds to enable them to finish the season so disastrously cut short." '

The Metropolitan Streets Act of 1867 showed Parliament what concerted action could do to control rabies — especially when backed by adequate legal sanctions, but Britain was comparatively slow in eradicating or even controlling rabies by controlling the movement of animals. In 1874 seventy-four people died from hydrophobia in Britain, almost half a century after Norway and Sweden had successfully contained the spread of rabies by controlling dogs. Under the powers of the Rabies Order of 1887 magistrates were enabled to make muzzling and leashing orders for the control of rabies in their areas. This had little effect because of dog-owners' firm dislike of muzzling. In 1897 an Act of Parliament gave the police all over the country the same powers as the Metropolitan Police to apprehend and destroy stray dogs. The importation of dogs and cats was controlled. Animals could only be imported under licence and had to spend six months in quarantine before being permitted to join their owners. These measures led to the disappearance of rabies from Britain by 1903. Inevitably, though, after the First World War at least one returning serviceman illegally imported a dog which was incubating rabies, and started an outbreak in Scotland which spread to Southern England.

Role of wildlife

It is remarkable, in a country as well stocked with foxes as England in the nineteenth century (and no doubt earlier), that foxes and other wildlife did not become infected with rabies. Admittedly, there is little

9

reason to suppose that foxes ever search out the company of dogs; and certainly any fox hunted by a pack of hounds containing some early sufferers from the disease would not survive to incubate the infection once the pack caught up with it, but, despite these observations, it is difficult to understand why, in the long history of rabies in Britain, carnivorous wildlife seems never to have been involved.

The epizootiology of rabies, although superficially straightforward, is not as simple as it seems. Although the disease is commonly spread to new hosts by the bite of an infected animal this need not always be so, as we shall see later. Even where the bite route is overwhelmingly important in the transfer of infected saliva, each region or country which has been closely studied shows an individual picture different in important particulars from others. The ecology of rabies virus may be divided, fairly arbitrarily, into urban and sylvatic phases. Almost everywhere the urban phase implicates domestic animals, especially dogs; the sylvatic, wildlife — the species of animals involved depending upon the locality. The urban and sylvatic phases may overlap, and in some places the overlap which occurs is of great significance in the maintenance of rabies; in others, as in Britain, the overlap is of no immediate significance but is potentially very important. Despite the fact that in many parts of the world the epizootiology of this terrifying disease has been rather fully worked out, there are, nevertheless, many problems which still have no solutions and many observations which still do not fit the general picture. Clearly, this must be because the picture is in many ways incomplete and inaccurate, and requires thorough ecological investigation to clarify it. Even so, enough is known in many parts to enable the disease to be combated rationally.

Hydrophobia in man has historically been related mainly to the incidence of rabies in dogs. As a result little attention was generally paid to the occurrence of rabies in wildlife unless, as in the epizooty in foxes in Switzerland and Southern Germany from 1803 to about 1835, the involvement of wild animals was so marked as to obtrude on the notice of even the dullest observer. Now, however, the importance of wild animals in the maintenance and spread of the infection is seriously studied and widely accepted. The authors of this book are all interested in European rabies since it is from the Continent that the infection will almost certainly come if it does indeed become established in Britain. Nevertheless, we have no doubt that the study of the disease in other parts of the world is valuable; the more that is known about an enemy, the more effectively can his moves be countered.

The United States of America is probably the continental area most thoroughly investigated regarding all aspects of the epizootiology of rabies. In the United States human deaths from rabies are now rare — about one per year, on average. This fortunate circumstance is almost entirely due to repeated effective campaigns to vaccinate dogs against the disease. Although rabies in dogs is now almost as rare in the United States as rabies in man, the disease continues to exist and flourish, with very little direct impingement on man.

Rabies in the United States is today pre-eminently a disease of wildlife. Despite the fact that every warm-blooded animal is susceptible to infection with rabies virus, in each situation there is usually one species which is epidemiologically the most important. In the United States the epidemiologically important species are different in different regions. In the eastern part of the country, bounded by the Appalachian Mountains on the west, it is the fox which supports the circulation of the virus and hence the maintenance of the disease. This is *Vulpes vulpes*, the familiar red fox of Europe and Britain. The animal has an extensive range in the New World, being found not only in the eastern United States but throughout sub-arctic Canada. Further west, on the prairie, the most important host is the spotted skunk (*Spilogale putorius*). This was the 'phoby cat' of the cowboys in the early years of the West. The presence of 'phoby cats' during the pioneer days suggests that rabies was not a new or recent infection in these parts, but one which had been established for a long time. Further south, in Florida and parts of Louisiana, raccoons are increasing in importance as a reservoir and source of rabies virus. In the Rocky Mountain states and California the striped skunk (*Mephitis mephitis*) and ground squirrels are the wild animals most heavily affected.

A particular species may be ecologically the most important in a region, but this does not exclude other species from the risk of infection and even some importance as carriers of the virus. Since 1953 when rabies virus was first isolated from insectivorous bats in Florida and Pennsylvania, the number of states reporting the presence of rabies in bats increased steadily until 1967 when all forty-eight continental states of the Union had done so. Many of the early isolations were made from the Mexican free-tailed bat (*Tadarida brasiliensis*), but many other species have yielded virus. The free-tailed bat is particularly important in Texas and New Mexico where immense populations are found. The epidemiological importance of insectivorous bats in the overall picture of rabies is difficult to assess. Bats undoubtedly infect each other in their roosts, and there are a few well-established examples of bats infecting men or other animals. There are, however, no observations to support a belief that insectivorous bats are of more than very minor importance as vectors (or carriers) of rabies to terrestrial mammals.

The discovery of bat rabies in the United States did lead, however, to the further discovery that the bite route — the direct implantation

11

of infected saliva into the tissues of the new victim — is not the only natural route of infection. During the early investigation of rabies in bats samples were taken of animals roosting in caves. Despite strict precautions against bites by bats during this work one of the workers went down with an encephalitis — an inflammation of the brain — which was diagnosed as rabies, from which he died. Since the bite route was excluded experiments were set up to test the possibility of infection by two other mechanisms: transfer of virus by insects and direct infection by the aerial route (i.e. breathing in the virus). Animals ranging in size from mice to foxes were housed in insect-proof cages and put around the caves in areas where there was considerable activity by bats. One after another the 'sentinel' animals sickened and died; rabies virus was isolated from the brains of all of them. The dust on the floor of the caves was subsequently found to be quite heavily contaminated with rabies virus which reached it in the saliva and urine of the bats roosting above. Bats may therefore be infected, not only during fights in the roosting place, but also by breathing in contaminated dust. It is also possible that terrestrial mammals such as coyotes may acquire the infection the same way when they enter the caves, and thus in their turn become vectors.

There was much interest in the source of infection of the insectivorous bats. Free-tailed bats are migratory and fly south for the winter. Ecological investigation has established that the southern part of the range of migrating free-tailed bats overlaps the northern range of at least one of the two commonest species of vampire bats which are haematophagous or blood eating — *Desmodus rufus* and *D. rotundus*. Unlike most species of bats, vampires do not have settled roosts to which they always return, but are gregarious and tend to roost where they find other bats. Since vampires are known to be able to feed on sleeping birds and human beings without even awakening them it is not difficult to imagine an infected vampire bat transferring virus to a roosting companion of another species. In any event, because bats tend to be quarrelsome creatures other possibilities for the transfer of infection exist.

In Central America and large areas of South America vampire bats are extremely important in the epidemiology of rabies of terrestrial mammals, unlike the situation in the United States where insectivorous bats are probably of minor or even negligible importance. The disease caused by rabies virus from vampires (and also other bats) is usually, if not always, of the type known as paralytic (see Chapters 3 & 4). This may indicate a biological difference in bat strains as compared with dog or fox strains of virus. Not enough experimental work has been done on the comparison of virus strains to make this more than an interesting idea. In those Central and Southern American countries with vampire bats as part of their fauna, fatal paralysis of cattle by bat-induced rabies-virus infection causes heavy economic loss. *Desmodus rotundus* is found from Mexico to Northern Argentina and losses of cattle in the same area have been estimated at between 500 000 and 1 000 000 head per year. Vampires seem to prefer bovine blood to most other sorts. In an outbreak of fatal paralytic disease afterwards shown to be rabies, human beings in rural Trinidad sleeping out of doors on verandahs were attacked and infected only where the cattle were enclosed in sheds at night to protect them from vampire attacks. The great majority of human cases of rabies in South America are caused by dog bites. It is not known whether a terrestrial animal infected by a vampire may become the source of an entirely terrestrial epizooty, but the possibility is worth investigating.

There have been several reports of the isolation of rabies virus from bats in Europe. Some of these isolates, especially those from Yugoslavia and Turkey, are fairly certainly rabies-related viruses of the sort discussed in Chapter 2. The German isolates, however, are difficult to explain. If, as I think we may safely do, we exclude Transylvanian vampires of the genus Dracula, there are no known haematophagous bats in Europe. There is therefore, no mechanism in Europe by which rabies virus could readily be transferred to insectivorous bats. The question of rabies in European bats clearly needs more work; but I believe that bats are unlikely to be a serious danger as vectors of rabies in Europe.

It is seldom easy to establish a clear link between wildlife rabies and rabies maintained by serial infection of dogs. In the western United States inquisitive dogs will probably, from time to time, be bitten by skunks, with a reasonable likelihood that sooner or later a biting skunk will be rabid. In South Africa where the situation is superficially similar the outcome is different. Rabies in the central part of the country – the northern Cape Province and the Orange Free State – is carried mainly if not entirely in the yellow mongoose and the meerkat. Occasionally human beings, usually children, are bitten by a rabid meerkat or mongoose, develop rabies, and die. In this large area of South Africa dog rabies is rare. The eastern part of the country, however, especially Zululand and Natal, recently experienced dog rabies, and the circulation of virus seemed to be confined entirely to dogs. This outbreak was an extension of an epizooty of dog rabies in Mozambique which lies immediately north of Zululand. Rabies is present in the whole of Africa and is occasionally reported in wild animals such as hyenas, but wherever the disease involves man the most likely vector, with few exceptions, is the dog. An adequate investigation of the ecology of rabies virus in Africa would almost certainly show the involvement of wildlife. Only such an investigation would be able to define a link between wildlife and dog rabies.

In India the incidence of human infection is, in absolute numbers, large, although it is not known with any great accuracy. Jackals, which carry rabies, and dogs, which are the main source for man, not infrequently meet and transact business on urban middens. In large cities like Delhi I have often seen them scavenging side by side and fighting on rubbish dumps. This may well have a special significance for Britain where foxes are found with increasing frequency as urban scavengers (see Chapter 6).

During the centuries that rabies was present in Britain before it was eradicated in 1903, and again in 1922, there is no evidence that the disease maintained itself in any animals other than dogs and sometimes cats. Rabies in wildlife did not exist, or·if it did, went unrecognized. Had there been a reservoir of virus in British wildlife, however, rabies would certainly not have been eradicated. We must accept therefore, that, for whatever reason, rabies failed to become established in British wildlife. Any re-importation in a dog or cat of rabies which is uncontrolled for long enough may lead to the establishment of sylvatic rabies. When rabies was imported in one smuggled dog in 1919 more than 200 dogs were infected; the contaminated areas spread from Scotland to southern England, and it took three years for the disease to be eradicated once more. The British countryside has undergone major changes in the fifty-five years since that episode was ended; the ecology of foxes has changed with the extension of their range of habitats to towns (see Chapter 6), and nobody can now safely say that sylvatic rabies is unlikely to occur in Britain because it was not known in the two previous exposures of the country to the disease.

The post-war European experience points very clearly to the red fox being the most important factor in the epidemiology of rabies on the Continent. Very soon after the Second World War veterinary authorities became aware of a wave of rabies advancing westwards across Europe. It is an interesting speculation that the movement of armies, the destruction of ecosystems, and the unrestrained growth of the fox population may have set the epizooty of the post-war years going just as the upheavals of the Napoleonic Wars may have been instrumental in permitting the outbreak in European foxes which flourished until 1835 or later. The geographical course of the present epizooty differs from that of the early nineteenth century which seemed to start in the Jura region and then spread westwards and northwards. The present epizooty came from the east. Rabid foxes moved from Poland to East Germany in 1948 and travelled across the north German plain until by 1950 the disease was present in West Germany and began spreading northwards through Schleswig-Holstein towards Denmark. In northern Germany many cattle were infected by foxes and farmers suffered considerable economic loss. The virus entered Denmark and advanced steadily northwards through Jutland; it was stopped and excluded from Denmark only by strenuous measures to control the fox population. When fox control was slackened rabies returned, brought by foxes from Schleswig-Holstein. Denmark is now kept free from rabies by the maintenance of a fox-free zone north of the border with Germany. Keeping the zone free of foxes requires a permanent effort since foxes tend to enter it from both sides to take advantage of the vacant territory.

From the northern part of the Federal German Republic the virus was carried southward through Hesse to Baden-Württemberg and westwards and southwards to Westphalia and the Rhineland. In these *Lände* the disease has been controlled, but not eradicated, by controlling the fox populations. The authorities discovered by practical experience that they need not exterminate foxes to keep a particular area free of rabies. When the fox population was reduced to less than one per square km rabies died away in that area. It was thought that at such a low population density the chance of foxes meeting and transferring disease-causing agents, including rabies virus, is reduced sufficiently to make the further propagation of rabies virus very improbable. The eological contributions to this book – Chapters 5 and 6 – indicate that simple descriptions are not always adequate.

The control of fox populations by slaughter may have been successful in controlling rabies in some circumstances, but the French experience shows rather clearly that it does not always do so. Rabies invaded France from Germany in 1968 and at first made only modest advances. The map shows how the disease spread during the next $7\frac{1}{2}$ years – and this in the face of a vigorous programme of fox control. Although the average rate of movement of rabies in France is about 80 km per year where it has moved fastest, there are places where it has averaged only about 12 km per year (see Chapter 6). The map shows clearly that the rate has fluctuated widely from year to year in any particular sector. It is therefore not wise to predict the expected movement in any year either by extrapolating from the previous year's distance or from the average distance over several years. This unwisdom is emphasized by looking at predictions: at slow rates of movement it could take as long as fifteen years for rabies to reach the Channel ports; at the fastest rates it may well get there by the summer of 1978.

The Channel is a moat wide enough and deep enough to keep rabies from Britain unless an animal incubating the disease is carried across, either accidentally or because somebody has deliberately smuggled it into the country. In either event the Ministry of Agriculture, Fisheries, and Food would set its contingency plans in operation (see Chapters

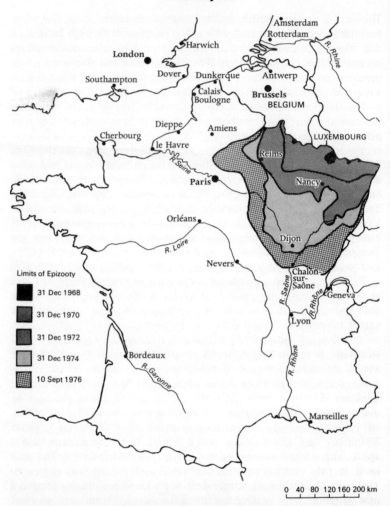

This map on the spread of rabies throughout France, was redrawn from one kindly supplied by Dr. Louis Andral, Directeur de la Centre d'Etudes de Rage, Malzeville, Nancy, France.

5 and 6). It would be unable to do this, however, until the first recognized case advertized an incipient outbreak.

I believe that long-term control of rabies in Europe, and other geographical areas where the involvement of wildlife has been studied and is reasonably well understood, will depend on successful efforts to immunize the most important vector animals against the disease.

The world problem

This is a general approach which has been successful in many other communicable diseases; and, indeed, has been successfully applied to dog rabies in many countries. Dogs, it is true, are easier to find and to immunize than foxes, but as Turner points out in Chapter 7 the problems associated with vaccinating foxes are being investigated with a reasonable probability of solving them.

The solution of the fox rabies problem would not necessarily mean the end of the rabies epizooty. Other biting animals may take the place of the fox. For various reasons it is unlikely that the smaller carnivores among the mustelids — stoats and weasels — would do so, but rabid polecats, martens and badgers might become more common. At present mustelids, badgers especially, tend to become infected because a fox or a family group of foxes may have made its den in a badger's set. A possible successor to the fox is the raccoon dog (*Nyctereutes procyonoides*). This fox-like animal was introduced from eastern Asia into European Russia. It has extended its range so far into Sweden, Poland and eastern Germany. Its potential as a vector of rabies should not be disregarded.

Rabies is, after all, a communicable disease which, as it is investigated more thoroughly, conforms more closely to a general pattern than was once thought. When an infectious-disease agent enters a community the extent to which it spreads depends on the degree of immunity in that community. Subjects with demonstrable immunity to a given agent will withstand infection by it; those without immunity will be susceptible and, if infected, may develop the disease, when the outcome will be either death or recovery. Recovered subjects will be immune to re-infection. A proportion of those infected may not show any signs of disease but develop immunity nevertheless. Thus, during the course of an epidemic prevalence of a disease the number of susceptibles diminishes until there are too few to support the transmission of the agent. The epidemic therefore ends, and the agent cannot re-establish itself in that community until the number of susceptibles increases. This may be partly by immigration, but is mainly by the accretion of new entrants by birth. An admirable example of this sort of history of an epidemic is offered by measles in an unvaccinated population of children.

Although 100 per cent mortalities have been reported for some communicable diseases in very special circumstances, such a clean sweep is rare. Even the most virulent strains of myxomatosis virus did not kill every rabbit. It is not surprising to learn, therefore, that despite its reputation as a killing agent rabies virus may behave in much the same way as more 'normal' communicable disease agents. In parts of the world where foxes, for example, are involved in the spread of rabies, it has been found that about 3 per cent of the animals tested have antibody to rabies virus in their blood. The implication of this finding is that at least a few foxes survive the infection. It is not known whether or not these animals may become carriers of the virus. Before such a theory could be seriously entertained a mechanism would have to be demonstrated whereby a latent infection suppressed by immunity would be reactivated. Such experiments have been made in guinea pigs and other small animals, and latent rabies virus may, indeed, be reactivated in these animals. This does not, of course, mean that foxes are also subject to reactivated rabies infection; but it does provide grounds for a well-planned investigation.

The part, if any, played by defective interfering particles of rabies virus (see Chapter 2) in latent and inapparent infections has still to be determined. Much work remains to be done in this field, but because it is expensive in both time and money it may not be tackled on a sufficiently large scale to ensure valid results in the reasonably near future.

Recent work in northern Argentina has shown that populations of vampire bats apparently respond to rabies virus in the same way that other hosts respond to other infectious agents. Many individuals in the population are infected. Some die; others survive the infection and anti-body can be demonstrated in their blood. In time the disease disappears from the population and does not return until there are once more enough susceptible bats in the population. There is thus a small but increasing amount of evidence that rabies virus is, in its epidemiological behaviour, not greatly different from what might loosely be called the general run of infectious agents.

If this is so, then the problem of rabies becomes, paradoxically, both simpler and more complex. Simpler in the sense that it falls more or less neatly into line with other infectious diseases about which we know quite a lot; more complex because the question of symptomless carriers of the virus must be looked at more seriously than most people have done up to now. Apparently healthy, symptomless dogs have been reported to cause rabies by their bites. L. Andral showed in 1957, while at the Pasteur Institute, Addis Ababa, that some of the stray dogs collected from the town had antibody to rabies virus in their blood; he was unable, for technical reasons, to determine whether these dogs were infected but symptomless, or had recovered from the disease. Nonetheless, the simple fact of the demonstration was of great importance, despite the fact that it caused little stir at the time.

There is, however, at least one well-documented account of a symptomless canine transmitter of infectious rabies virus. This, the case of the dog from Surandai, was reported by Dr N. Veeraraghavan, then the Director of the Pasteur Institute of Southern India, Coonoor. After a case of hydrophobia which followed the bite of an apparently healthy dog at Surandai (a village not far from Coonoor) the dog was identified, removed to the Institute and kept in isolation in the Institute's compound. During the first five months that it was observed rabies virus was isolated from thirteen different samples of its saliva. Subsequently one more isolation was made a year after the dog was taken to the Institute; but this was after a course of cortico-steroid hormone which tends to inhibit the body defences which prevent latent infections from becoming apparent. When the dog died after slightly more than three years at the Institute, without ever having shown symptoms of rabies, its brain and spinal cord were thoroughly investigated. No infectious virus was isolated, but the presence of some structural material or virus antigen (see Chapter 2) was demonstrated by immunofluorescent microscopy.

Clearly, more investigations should be made into the possibility that symptomless canine carriers of rabies may exist. This information could be very important in studies of the epidemiology of the disease. A further important aspect of the case is that it suggests that infection of the nervous system by rabies virus may not always be fatal; but until confirmed by more thoroughly investigated cases this is no more than a supposition. It is also important to investigate the dangers of reactivation of the possibly latent infection in foxes found with circulating antibody to rabies virus.

There appears to be another situation in which rabies virus may cause an inapparent or latent infection. Several Central European virologists have reported the isolation of 'rabies-like' viruses from small field rodents such as the common vole (*Microtus arvalis*), the yellow-necked mouse (*Apodemus flavicollis*), and the wood mouse (*A. sylvaticus*). The first group of these isolations was reported from Czechoslovakia by A. Sodja in 1969. Some of the animals from which virus was isolated were trapped in parts of the country where rabies was active in foxes, but others were taken in an area where rabies had not been reported for twenty years or more. About 2 per cent of Sodja's trapped animals yielded 'rabies-like' virus. Sodja's findings were confirmed in West Germany by L.G. Schneider, who also reported that about 2 per cent of his animals carried the virus. Scheider made a thorough serological investigation of the antigens of his isolates, and some of Sodja's, by comparing their reactions with antibodies made by immunizing rabbits against each isolate, and with antibodies against a 'standard' rabies virus and rabies virus from foxes. He included in his comparison some of the rabies-related viruses (see Chapter 2) and, in short, tested each virus strain against each antibody preparation. It is necessary to test for so-called reciprocal cross-reactions in this way to determine the closeness of any relationships which may exist in the group of antigens being investigated. As a result of his tests Schneider decided that the viruses that he and Sodja had isolated were not sufficiently different from authentic rabies virus strains to justify the rather cautious and non-committal name given them by Sodja. He therefore called them rabies viruses of rodent origin.

Professor F. Steck of the Institute of Veterinary Microbiology, University of Bern, isolated similar viruses from voles captured in northern Switzerland. He could not repeat the isolation of his first strain when he retested the original vole material with stringent precautions. He remained sceptical, therefore, of the significance of the isolation because he was unable to convince himself that he had not inadvertently contaminated his vole material with rabies virus previously handled in his laboratory. This sort of contamination has occurred not infrequently in work with other viruses, and has only relatively recently been recognized as a very likely risk in a busy laboratory handling several viruses. However, both Sodja and Schneider are confident of the reliability of their work.

It is difficult to find a place for rabies virus of rodent origin in the epidemiology of the disease as it has been worked out in Central and Western Europe. The amount of virus present in those voles or mice giving positive tests seems to be very small, and voles are among the most highly susceptible animals. Isolations of virus are made by injecting suspensions of organs of captured animals into the brains of laboratory mice. The inoculated mice must then be observed very closely for the slightest sign of abnormality; if they are not killed when this occurs they recover, and subsequently no trace of an infecting virus can be found. However, when such a slightly abnormal mouse is killed and a suspension of its brain inoculated, in turn, into the brain of a fresh mouse, the second mouse develops more definite symptoms. The process is repeated in series in the laboratory (it is called 'passaging') and by the third or fourth passage the amount of virus has been amplified sufficiently to kill the test mouse. The rather slow amplification of virus which seems to be occurring may, possibly, indicate that the incompletely understood phenomenon of virus adaptation is taking place. With many viruses of animals, when a virus is transferred to a host of a different species it fails to do to the new host what it did regularly in the previous one. When the virus (or an extract of its presumed target tissue or organ) is passaged serially in individuals of the new species, adaptation is shown by the new species eventually developing the appropriate signs of infection. The basic phenomenon is probably the selection of mutants of the original virus which are more virulent for the new host than the original was (see Chapter 4).

When rabies virus is transferred to a new host species by injection into the central nervous system (i.e. the brain) it does not need a period of adaptation to enable it to kill the new host. What does happen, however, is that the incubation period before the onset of symptoms is of variable length, but during serial passage in the new host species the incubation period becomes shorter and is eventually fixed at so many days with a range of about one day each side. When Pasteur transferred virus from a rabid dog to rabbits, the incubation period in rabbits of the *virus des rue* (or 'street' virus) was both long and variable. Eventually, however, the incubation period became shorter and more regular at about 6 to 8 days. Pasteur called the virus thus adapted to rabbits *virus fixe* (or 'fixed' virus). Thus, if the virus as it occurs in voles and other field rodents does need to undergo 'adaptation' to laboratory mice, it is unlikely to be of much, or indeed any consequence in the epizootiology of rabies, since it is impossible to envisage an adequate passage series from voles through foxes or other predators. If, however, the process of isolating these viruses from voles is simply an amplification of a minute amount of virus present in the brain or brown fat it is possible that exposure of the carrier voles in their natural habitat to appropriate stimuli may cause a latent infection to become apparent. A vole with such an activated infection would presumably act as a focus of infection for the population of which it was part; and, since field voles are among the animals most highly susceptible to rabies, an epizooty would occur in the voles. Many voles would die, but many would be available sources of virus for the infection of predators feeding on them. Neither of these theoretical possibilities (activated latent infection and infection of predators feeding on infected voles) has been tested experimentally, which would be very difficult to do convincingly. If, however, such viruses were isolated from field rodents in Britain, where not only has sylvatic rabies apparently been unknown, but where not even dog rabies has existed for more than fifty years, then it would be clear that whatever the consequences to those rodents which carry them, they are of no consequence in the epizootiology of rabies. Such a study is at present being made as part of an ecological investigation of virus carriage in British field rodents.

If rabies virus is imported into Britain in a smuggled animal during the incubation of its infection, and if the animal, when symptoms develop, is not recognized for what it is, then it is probable that the disease will be able to establish itself. The virus would certainly circulate in dogs and very likely in cats, too. A rabid cat almost invariably develops the furious form of the disease and is able to inflict severe and dangerous wounds often on a dismayingly large number of victims. Macdonald (Chaper 6) points out the potential danger to foxes of rabid cats.

The best defence against rabies in Britain is clearly to keep it out. The recent Rabies Act, with its very severe penalties for the unlicensed, illegal landing of prescribed animals in Britain is the best defense we have. But even the best laws are not proof against dishonesty or human stupidity.

2
Rabies virus

F. BROWN and J. CRICK

During the last decade the physical and chemical properties of viruses have been used increasingly as a basis for their classification. One of the most important and fundamental characteristics of a virus particle is its shape, and rabies virus belongs to a group of viruses which are described as bullet-shaped or bacilliform. These viruses are called rhabdoviruses (from rhabdos, the Greek word for rod) and more than sixty of them have been found in many different kinds of host. For example, there are rhabdoviruses in plants (e.g. plantain virus, potato yellow dwarf virus), insects (e.g. Sigma virus), fish (e.g. infectious haematopoietic necrosis virus), birds (e.g. Flanders and Hart Park viruses) and animals (e.g. rabies virus and vesicular stomatitis virus). Some of the viruses multiply in more than one kind of host (e.g. vesicular stomatitis virus and potato yellow dwarf virus will also replicate in insects), and indeed one of the features of the rhabdoviruses is their wide host range.

Rabies virus is able to infect all warm-blooded animals. During the last ten to fifteen years it has been shown to have a highly complex structure. The fundamental characteristics of this structure have been worked out but much remains to be done. In this chapter we relate the structural features of the virus, as they are known at present, to its biological properties. The relationship of rabies virus to the recently described rabies-related viruses is also considered. Finally, the way in which the virus multiplies and the importance of defective virus particles in this process are also described.

Structural Features

Morphology
The main structural features of rabies virus were first ascertained by electron microscopy of thin sections of cells infected with the virus, but details of the structure have been obtained from preparations of the purified virus particles themselves. Examination of thin sections of chick-embryo or baby-hamster-kidney cells infected with the virus first indicated the association of infectivity with the bullet-shaped

particles. Bullet-shaped particles 140 X 100 nanometres (nm) long with surface projections about 6 nm long were seen. (A nanometre is one millionth part of a millimetre.) A vesicular appendage at the flat end of the particles, a central channel and a helical ribbon-like structure emanating from some of the particles were seen in the infected cells. The similarity of these particles to the well-characterized vesicular stomatitis virus was noted.

More detailed examination of the purified particles showed that they appeared to consist of an internal helical structure (the ribonucleo-protein), surrounded by a closely associated protein layer (the matrix), the two structures together forming the core or 'skeleton' of the particle. The skeleton was surrounded in turn by a membranous envelope which was covered on its surface by fine projections extending about 10 nm from it. The virus also had a well-defined honeycomb-like structure which probably reflects a symmetry in underlying layers (see below).

When the stain used in electron microscopy penetrates the virus particles the envelope layer can be seen as a three-layered membrane. More extensive penetration of the stain reveals transverse cross striations of the internal helix, similar to those found in vesicular stomatitis virus. In rabies virus the helix has thirty to thirty-five coils in the form of a cylinder 50 nm wide and about 150 nm long. When the virus particles break spontaneously or after addition of a mild detergent, the internal helix is released as a loosely coiled ribbon. A model of the virus particle has recently been proposed by Vernon and his colleages.

Other virus-like particles are also found in harvests from cells infected with rabies virus. Most prominent among these are bullet-shaped particles which have the same morphological features as the virus particles but are about one third the length. These particles, which can be separated readily from the full-length virus particles, have been shown to interfere with virus growth. Their importance in the replication of the virus is considered more fully below.

Long virus particles, up to two to three times the length of the normal virus particles, are also found. As with the short particles, the general morphological features are similar to those of the normal length particles.

Chemistry

Until recently large amounts of rabies virus could be grown only in the brains of experimental animals. Purification of this virus was both difficult and inadequate. The application of modern tissue-culture techniques has meant that enough material can now be made available for detailed physico-chemical analysis. The virus grows to fairly high concentrations in cultures of suitable cells, and is set free in the medium, causing little structural damage to the cells. This means that it can be concentrated and purified from such tissue-culture fluids free

23

from gross contamination by cellular debris. This is important for chemical studies. By addition of appropriate radioactive substances to the nutrient medium during the growth of the virus it is possible to obtain virus with a radioactive label in its nucleic acid or in any other chemical component.

Several methods are available for the purification of the virus. The one we have mainly used depends on precipitation of the virus by addition of a salt (e.g. zinc acetate or ammonium sulphate) to reduce the volume of material to be handled. The precipitated virus is re-suspended in a suitable volume and subjected to high speed centrifugation to sediment it to a pellet at the bottom of the tube. The pellet is re-suspended in a small volume and subjected once more to centrifugation, but this time in a solution of sucrose of increasing density from the top of the tube to the bottom. This is known as centrifugation in a sucrose gradient. It is an extremely powerful method, widely used in biochemistry and virology, which separates molecules and particles according to size and shape, and at the same time introduces a very considerable purification factor. After this centrifugation a visible band of virus is seen in the tube. In some infected cell cultures defective interfering particles are also produced. Because they are smaller and less dense than complete virus particles the visible band is nearer the top of the tube than the complete virus particles.

Purified rabies virus particles contain about two per cent to three per cent ribonucleic acid (RNA) and some carbohydrate; more than half of each particle consists of protein and about a quarter of lipid.

The RNA, which carries the genetic information necessary for the production of more virus particles by infected cells, is not, when analysed by the usual chemical methods, readily distinguishable from the RNA of other rhabdoviruses.

Proteins are an important part of any biological system. Modern methods of analysis are simple, rapid, and elegant, and depend upon a process called electrophoresis. In this process the proteins of the virus are separated from each other and caused to move in an electrical field. The process is confined within a rod of gelatinous material and is therefore known as electrophoresis in gel. Molecules move in an electrophoretic field at rates which vary with their size (molecular weight) and charge, but in the presence of a mild detergent the rate of movement depends almost entirely on their molecular weight. By comparison with the final positions in the gel of proteins of known molecular weight, the molecular weights of proteins under test can be determined. Rabies virus contains four major proteins, each of different molecular weight, and one minor protein (proteins G, N, M_1, M_2, and L). The number of copies of each protein in a virus particle can be calculated by relating the amount of each protein at its final position in the gel to its molecular weight. The location of the different proteins in the virus is discussed below.

Not much is known about the carbohydrate and lipid of rabies virus, but it is known that the G protein contains carbohydrate, and that there is some carbohydrate in the lipid fraction of the membrane of the virus. Lipid is found only in the outer membrane of the virus and has a composition somewhat different from that of the bounding or plasma membrane of the cells in which the virus was grown. This has certain implications which are discussed in the section on the replication of the virus in infected cells.

Structural sub-units and their biological activities

The presence of lipid in the outer coat of rabies virus particles makes it relatively easy to disrupt them simply by the addition of a lipid solvent such as ether, or by mixing them with a mild detergent. The products can then be examined in the electron microscope and separated from each other by different physical methods. By analysing the different fragments by electrophoresis in gel, the proteins associated with each structure can then be determined and in this way a model of the virus can be built up.

Treating the virus with the detergent Nonidet P40, for example, removes the lipid and the surface glycoproteins, leaving a skeleton-like structure. The great difference in size of the glycoprotein molecules and the skeleton allows them to be separated easily by centrifugation. Similarly, treatment of the virus with a bile salt, sodium deoxycholate, releases the ribonucleic acid as a string-like structure (the ribonucleoprotein) in which it is in close association with the single protein, N. A model of the virus which has biological significance starts to emerge when the different fragments are also tested for their biological activity.

The surface projections consist of a glycoprotein (protein G). This protein, which is presumed to be important in the attachment of the virus to susceptible cells, also carries the antigen which elicits the production of neutralizing antibody when inoculated into animals, and hence affords protection against the disease. Moreover, the antigenic specificity of the virus (see Chapter 1, p.4) is located on the glycoprotein. This means that the antigenic difference between the classical rabies virus and the rabies-related viruses (see below) is associated with the spikes.

Rabies virus agglutinates red blood cells — i.e. it makes them stick together — and this activity also is associated with the glycoprotein. In contrast to the ability of the glycoprotein to stimulate in animals the production of neutralizing antibody even after its removal from the virus particle, the isolated glycoprotein does not agglutinate red blood cells.

This activity appears to depend on the integrity of the virus envelope.

On the other hand, the N protein of the ribonucleoprotein molecule which makes up the helical structure appears to be group-specific. When the ribonucleoprotein is inoculated into animals it stimulates production of antibody which reacts in tests like complement fixation and immunofluorescence (see Chapter 1, p.4) with the ribonucleoprotein molecules of other rabies-like viruses.

The reactions of the different proteins of the virus with their specific antibodies can be readily detected when the antibody is labelled with a fluorescent dye. This makes it easier to detect the presence of virus antigens in infected tissues and, because of this, the fluorescent antibody binding test is used extensively in diagnosis (see Chapter 1, p.4). By using the different specificites of the G and N proteins it is possible to distinguish between the type-specific reaction for which G is responsible and the group reaction, in which the N protein is involved.

The other two major proteins M_1 and M_2 are thought to be the proteins concerned with the organization of the ribonucleoprotein strand into its helical configuration and subsequently into the membrane of the bullet-shaped particles. In their model of rabies virus, Vernon and his colleagues have depicted the larger of the two M proteins (M_1) as being adjacent to the ribonucleoprotein. The smaller of the two M proteins (M_2) was considered to be closely associated with the virus lipids in lipoprotein aggregates or micelles and regarded as forming an integral part of the virus envelope.

The distinct honeycomb appearance of rabies virus in electron micrographs is probably due to an ordered arrangement of the protein sub-units, the glycoprotein molecules being arranged in a hexagonal pattern outside the micellar layer.

A minor protein (L) is also present in rabies virus, but its location and role are not known with any certainty. It has been considered, by analogy with vesicular stomatitis virus, to be associated with an enzyme for the replication of the ribonucleic acid of the virus. However, demonstration of such an enzyme activity has been difficult with rabies virus, and there is no certainty at this stage that such an enzyme is present in the particles.

Rabies-related viruses

Until recently, rabies virus was regarded as a serological entity unrelated to other members of the rhabdovirus group. Although isolates of rabies virus with different biological properties have been described, little antigenic variation was found between them, and it is standard practice to use the same strain throughout the world for the production of vaccines and antisera.

The concept of antigenic unity has been challenged recently by

Rabies virus

Shope and Murphy and their colleagues in the USA, who have shown that serological and morphological relatedness exists between rabies virus and six other viruses, two of which were first discovered about twenty years ago. The first, Lagos bat virus, was isolated from the brain of a frugivorous bat (*Eidolon helvam*) on Lagos Island, Nigeria, in 1956, and the second, Nigerian horse virus, was obtained in 1958 in Ibadan, Nigeria, from the brain of a horse which had died from 'staggers', a disease resembling rabies. The third and fourth members of the group, Obodhiang virus and kotonkan virus, are unusual among the rabies group of viruses in being insect-borne. Obodhiang virus was isolated in 1963 from pools of *Mansonia uniformis* mosquitoes in the Sudan, while kotonkan virus was obtained in 1967 from Culicoides midges in Nigeria. Three strains of the fifth virus, Mokola, were isolated in 1968 from the viscera of shrews (*Crocidura* sp.) captured in Ibadan, Nigeria, and, in the same area, two isolates were subsequently obtained from human beings. The sixth virus, Duvenhage, was found in South Africa in 1970 in the brain of a man who had died, apparently from rabies, after being bitten by a bat.

The interrelatedness of these viruses has been shown by complement fixation, neutralization, cross-protection, and fluorescent antibody tests. Nigerian horse virus is more like rabies virus than it is like Lagos bat or Mokola viruses. Obodhiang and kotonkan viruses are only distantly related to rabies virus, but more closely related to Mokola virus. In fact, recent comparative work from Yale University led Sonya Buckley to propose that Mokola virus is the biological and serological bridging agent within the group.

On the basis of serological tests it has been suggested that certain subdivisions within the rabies group can be made and that Lagos bat, Nigerian horse, and Mokola viruses should be regarded as new serotypes of rabies virus, so that classical rabies vaccines may not be effective against them. Tignor and Shope found that mice vaccinated with a rabies virus of reduced virulence were only poorly protected against Mokola virus. This was an important observation, since two strains of the latter were isolated from children, one of whom died. In addition, a case of laboratory infection with Mokola virus has occurred in Germany in an individual possessing a high concentration of neutralizing antibody against rabies virus.

As yet, we have little knowledge of the significance of the rabies-related viruses and whether they pose a threat to man or animals in certain parts of the world. Neither do we know whether these or other rabies-like viruses exist in the wild life of other countries. Antibodies to kotonkan virus have been found in human, cattle, rodent, and insectivore sera in northern Nigeria, and in cattle, sheep, and horse sera in the southern part of that country. Neutralization tests with sera

27

of cattle newly imported into Nigeria and suffering from a type of disease usually associated with bovine ephemeral fever virus, another rhabdovirus, suggest that kotonkan virus is the agent responsible. Studies of this virus show that it is morphologically similar to bovine ephemeral fever virus, both being cone-shaped, but there appears to be no serological relationship between ephemeral fever virus and any member of the rabies virus subgroup.

Shope and Tignor have suggested that a polyvalent vaccine or an appropriate combined vaccine regimen might be useful in certain areas such as West Africa in which more than one virus of the rabies group has been found, and the more recent isolation of Duvenhage virus in the Transvaal suggests that these considerations may apply equally to other parts of the African continent.

Replication of the virus

Under this heading we consider how the virus enters the cell, the synthesis of the virus components and their assembly, and, finally, how the completed virus is released. Since many of these studies have been made in tissue-culture cells we must remember that the events observed may not depict accurately what happens in an infected animal, particularly in nervous tissue for which rabies virus has a particular predilection.

Infection of the cell

It is widely accepted that many viruses are taken into cells by a process of engulfment or phagocytosis, although the alternative view is that, with viruses which possess lipoprotein envelopes, fusion may occur between the envelope and the cell membrane. Both processes have been observed in cultures of baby-hamster-kidney cells infected with rabies virus. In the first, virus particles passed into the cells and could be seen in cytoplasmic vesicles fifteen to thirty minutes after infection. Fusion of the virus envelope with plasma membranes and with the walls of phagocytic vacuoles has also been observed within minutes of infection, suggesting that after engulfment of the particle its envelope may fuse with cell membranes. The process of membrane fusion allows direct access of the virus genetic material (the genome) into the cell. The removal of the virus membrane is probably the most important step in uncoating since it exposes the nucleocapsid which is thought to contain the virus transcriptase, an enzyme necessary for the synthesis of copies of the RNA of the virus.

Synthesis of the virus components

Little is known directly of the method whereby rabies virus is reproduced in the infected cell. Investigations of this sort with viruses are generally made with the aid of radioactive tracer substances to label the RNA of the virus. Labelling of the cellular RNA in this type of experiment is prevented by treating the cells with the drug Actinomycin D. This is not possible with rabies virus because it grows so slowly that the drug would be in contact with the cells for long enough to kill them. Nevertheless, it is believed that the replication of rabies virus in infected cells is similar to that of vesicular stomatitis virus. If this is so, then the RNA and the various proteins which make up the virus are synthesized in various parts of the cytoplasm of the cells and are then assembled into nucleocapsids (i.e. the virus particle less its lipid membrane). The nucleocapsids attach to membranes, which have been converted into virus envelope by insertion of the G and M_2 proteins, to form complete particles, or virions as they are also called.

Virus maturation and release
The actual site of virus maturation and release from the cell is still a matter of debate. Traditionally, the formation of intracytoplasmic inclusions (Negri bodies or matrices), which are now know to be accumulations of ribonucleoprotein, were widely assumed to be an essential first step in virus maturation. The virus was thought to be completed at membranes formed *de novo* near the matrices and there was believed to be little budding from the cell surface. This idea was further substantiated by the fact that rabies virus remains largely associated with the cell, and by the discovery that the lipid content of rabies virus membranes was different from that of the plasma membranes of the cells from which the virus was derived. However, present consensus of opinion tends to the view that rabies virus particles may be formed either at the cell surface or associated with intracytoplasmic membranes, and need not be associated with the nucleoprotein inclusions at all. In fact, it has been suggested recently that these bodies may be formed only when there is a disarrangement of the process of virus maturation. Whether or not virus is released from the cell surface is thought to be determined more by the host cell itself than by the virus under study and budding has been observed at the surface of cells from tissues as diverse as salivary gland, muscle, and nervous tissue. Certainly budding from the plasma membranes, particularly in tissues such as salivary glands, would ensure the release of virus necessary for its transmission.

Other products from infected cells

In addition to infectious virus, a variety of other virus-induced products may be identified in harvests from cells infected with rabies virus. These may be examined by electron microscopy as described above or characterized by their serological or biological activities. The most important are probably rabies 'soluble' antigen, interferon, and defective particles.

Soluble antigen

The medium harvested from infected cells contains large quantities of non-infectious material with the immunological specificity of the G protein. This can be readily separated from the intact virions by centrifugation, and has the capacity to protect animals against challenge by virulent virus. It seems likely that the antigen is excess G protein which does not become incorporated into virus particles.

Interferon

In most cells infected with rabies virus, little or no specific damage is observed and the cells may be maintained in an actively growing state for long periods by regular division and feeding of the cultures. The maintenance of such a chronically infected state in baby-hamster-kidney cells has been attributed by workers at the Wistar Institute, Philadelphia, to the cyclic production of interferon, a protein produced by infected cells which interferes with virus growth. In their cell system, periodic cycles of low and high virus production appear to be related to the concentration of interferon in the culture. More recently, however, Matsumoto and his co-workers in Japan showed that in the same cells the establishment of persistent infection could be associated not with interferon but with the production of defective interfering particles (see below).

Defective particles

Shortened defective particles are produced by many rhabdoviruses. They are readily separated from the infectious particles in sucrose density gradients as described earlier, and usually have RNA only a quarter of the size of normal virus RNA. These particles are unable to replicate in the absence of the fully infective virus but interfere with its production. We have found that in cultures to which defective interfering particles had been added the yields of rabies virus were depressed by more than 99 per cent compared with controls. The interference seemed to be highly specific, for there was no effect on the replication of vesicular stomatitis virus.

Defective particles of both vesicular stomatitis virus and rabies virus appear to be associated with the development of persistently infected cells in cultures, yet in animals interference by defective interfering particles remains to be demonstrated satisfactorily. The first observations that interference may occur in animals infected with rabies virus were made more than twenty years ago by Koprowski and his colleagues. In a number of laboratories, including our own, it is not unusual for adult mice infected with very large doses of rabies virus, or one of the rabies-related viruses, to survive for long periods after infection, sometimes without overt disease. Some mice survive for many months in a semi-paralysed condition, or even recover completely. From time to time reports have appeared of dogs which have had abortive rabies, a condition reproduced experimentally by Dr J.F. Bell in the USA. There are accounts of animals developing rabies after exceptionally long incubation periods and readers may recall the case of the man from Bangladesh who died in Britain from rabies in 1976 after an incubation period of at least fourteen months. It is possible that interference may play a part in delayed or persistent infections, although there is as yet a lack of unequivocal evidence.

Summary

Recent research has shown that rabies virus is a bullet-shaped particle containing RNA, protein, lipid and carbohydrate. The RNA, which constitutes about 2 per cent of the particle, has a molecular weight of 4 million and codes for 4 major proteins and one minor protein. The function of two of these major proteins has been ascertained by dissecting the virus into biologically active subunits whose composition has been determined by electrophoresis in polyacrylamide gels. The spike projection consists of a single glycoprotein (G) which stimulates the production of neutralizing antibody and is responsible for the specific serological reactions of the virus. The nucleoprotein (N), on the other hand, is a group protein which cross reacts with antisera produced from the rabies-related viruses.

The rabies-related viruses which were discovered in Africa are closely related to rabies virus but differ sufficiently to allow them to be distinguished by serological tests. Moreover, animals protected against rabies virus are not necessarily immune to infection with the rabies-related viruses. The existence of these viruses thus presents a problem which should be considered in relation to vaccination against rabies in certain parts of Africa.

Rabies virus harvests also contain shortened defective interfering particles whose RNA is about one-quarter the length of that of the infective virus. These particles interfere with virus replication and may have a role in the establishment of slow or persistent infections.

3

Rabies in man

DAVID A. WARRELL

Definition

In man the disease called rabies is a severe inflammation of the brain and spinal cord (encephalomyelitis) associated with invasion of these tissues by rabies virus. It is virtually always fatal.

Importance of human rabies

About 700 human deaths due to rabies are reported to the World Health Organization each year, but this number is a gross underestimate of the true incidence. Most of the countries in which rabies is common are unable to obtain accurate statistics. Figures of 15 000 deaths each year for the whole world and 15 000 for India alone have been suggested. The Philippines has a population of about 32 million human beings and 3·7 million dogs. In 1964, 383 human beings and about 25 000 dogs died of rabies, an incidence in man of 1·2 per 100 000 population. These deaths occur despite the vaccination of 150 000 people each year ($\frac{1}{2}$ per cent of the population) following dog bites. These figures emphasize the medical importance of rabies in some parts of the world.

Rabies was eradicated from Britain by 1903. The last two patients to develop rabies after being infected in this country died in 1902, but there had been 173 deaths in England and Wales in the preceding 17 years. Between 1946 and 1976, 11 people who had been infected abroad died of rabies in England.

In all parts of the world rabies has a hold on the human imagination out of all proportion to its incidence. This is explained by the frightening and painful way in which the infection is spread to man — usually by a vicious bite from a mad dog — by the discomfort, risks, and uncertainties associated with traditional treatment after the bite; and by the unpredictable and sometimes very long incubation period before the disease declares itself. Dog-bite victims may have to endure a wait of several years before they can feel reasonably sure that they have escaped the threat of rabies. Finally, the disease itself is terrifying and

32

agonizing. Death after a few days of intense suffering is almost inevitable. Kuru is the only other communicable disease to share this hopeless outlook. This is a slow virus infection of the brain which is restricted to a cannibal tribe in New Guinea and is now almost extinct. Untreated sleeping sickness (African trypanosomiasis), which is still an important infection in parts of Africa, also approaches 100 per cent mortality, but many patients can be cured by drugs.

Routes of infection

Rabies infection in man is nearly always the result of a bite by an animal which has the virus in its saliva. Virus cannot penetrate unbroken skin but even a lick by an infected animal can be dangerous if the skin is grazed or damaged in some other way. Rabies virus can enter the body through the intact mucous membranes such as the conjunctival membrane covering the eye or the membranes lining the mouth, anus, and external genital organs. Laboratory animals can be infected by eating food containing the virus. This route has never been confirmed in man, but there have been several anecdotal reports including one from Charles Darwin in 1837.

Inhaling airborne rabies virus into the nose and throat is the rarest recorded route of infection in man. Only three cases are known. In 1956 and 1959 two men died of rabies after exploring Frio Caves in Uvalde County, Texas. These caves are inhabited by millions of insectivorous bats (Mexican free-tailed bats, *Tadarida brasiliensis mexicana*), about $\frac{1}{2}$ per cent of which are infected with rabies. The air in the caves held a fine suspension of rabies virus from the bats' saliva and urine. Both men denied being bitten by bats. They may have inhaled rabies virus or have been infected through breaks in their skin. In 1972 a veterinary surgeon died of rabies in the USA three weeks after grinding up rabid goat brain. He probably inhaled an aerosol of virus generated by the blending machine.

Post-vaccinal rabies is caused by injection of an antirabies vaccine which accidentally contains 'fixed' rabies virus which has not been properly killed. Fixed virus results from the repeated passage through experimental animals of the naturally-occurring 'street' virus (pp. 21 & 104). This makes it more predictable in its properties and more suitable for vaccine production. The virus used for human vaccines should be completely inactivated by chemicals such as phenol, but this has failed on a few occasions. In Fortaleza in Brazil in 1960 eighteen people died of an acute paralytic illness, four to thirteen days after being given their first injection of antirabies vaccine. Fixed virus was isolated from the brains of the victims and from the faulty batch of vaccine. Post-vaccinal fixed virus rabies resembles the paralytic form of rabies (see below) but has a shorter incubation period.

Theoretically, any warm blooded animal, including birds, could transmit rabies to man, but in fact more than 90 per cent of cases result from bites by the domestic dog. Cats are second in importance, followed by other domestic animals and wild animals.

Dog bite is a very common event in most parts of the world. In the USA $\frac{1}{2}$ per cent of the whole population is bitten each year, and as many as 15 per cent of children aged between two and ten years. In 1972 there were 38 000 animal bites, mostly by dogs, in New York City. In Britain the incidence of dog bites in one part of Liverpool was estimated as 500 per 100 000 people per year, and in Sunderland as 400 per 100 000 per year in children less than fifteen years old.

Bites by rabid dogs can be terribly destructive and disfiguring especially when they involve soft tissues such as the face. Children, being smaller and less able to defend themselves, are more likely to be bitten on the head than are adults.

Risks of infection and disease following bites

Assessment of the risk of developing the disease after a bite is one of the most difficult problems in the study of rabies. Unless the biting animal can be examined it is not possible to be certain whether the patient was even *exposed* to the risk of infection. If rabies virus is present in the saliva of the animal it can be assumed that the patient was *infected* (i.e. virus entered the body) but, even without any treatment, the patient may not develop rabies. The reason may be that insufficient numbers of virus particles were inoculated or that the body's own defences were able to inactivate the virus before it could get into a nerve and start its ascent to the brain.

The risk of developing the disease after infection increases with the severity of the bite. The greater the tissue damage the greater the chance of virus being able to enter nerves. Bites on the face carry the highest risk. The face has a rich nerve supply and its soft tissues are easily disrupted. Facial bites are associated with a very short incubation period, allowing less time for vaccine to stimulate the antibodies necessary to neutralize rabies virus before it can enter the nervous system.

If the bite wound made by a rabid animal is properly cleaned soon after the accident, and active and passive immunization are started, the risk of the virus reaching the central nervous system to cause clinical rabies can be reduced, perhaps tenfold.

Exposure, infection, and the clinical disease must not be confused. Each term implies a different risk of death and demands a different course of action. Examples of this confusion are two recent BBC news items. It was reported that a French rabies expert had recovered from the disease after being given vaccine, and that some British embassy personnel in Burma who had been bitten by a rabid dog had been given vaccine, 'even though they showed no signs of the disease'. In both cases there may have been infection with rabies but vaccine was given, in the first case successfully, to prevent clinical rabies, an inflammation of the central nervous system (encephalomyelitis) which is almost invariably fatal. A six-year-old boy was attacked by a rabid wolf in Iran in 1954. The wolf's fang penetrated the skull, tore through its tough membranous lining (dura mater), and entered the parietal lobe of the brain. Combined vaccine and antirabies serum was given by the Pasteur Institute and, despite the terrible injuries, rabies was prevented.

Some tragedies in Britain during the last few years have shown how easily a dog the size of an alsatian can kill a child, yet rabid animals very rarely kill people outright. This may be explained by a lack of persistence and sense of purpose in the frantic attacks by these sick animals.

Transmission of rabies from person to person

The saliva, tears, sputum, and other body secretions of human rabies victims contain rabies virus for about the first week of their illness. Since these patients may salivate, spit and cough over, or even bite the people near them, it is very surprising that person-to-person transmission of rabies is practically unknown. The older literature contains some anecdotal reports. The mother of Marcello Malpighi, the seventeenth-century pioneer microscopist, was bitten by her rabid daughter and died of rabies. In 1898 there occurred in Warsaw the unique case of a thirty-three-year-old man who caught rabies from his maidservant on the first day of her illness. Her saliva may have contaminated a small wound on his hand, but kissing or sexual intercourse might have been responsible for this transmission. Amongst 8600 people in contact with rabies victims under the care of the Pasteur Institutes during the 1930s only one developed rabies. More recently, in Laos, a man died of rabies after nursing a son who perished from the same disease. The possibility was, however, not excluded that the father had himself been bitten by a rabid animal. In fact, there is no completely documented case of man transmitting rabies to man. Attempts to resuscitate rabies patients and to prolong their lives by intensive care will increase the chances of medical staff becoming infected. As far as is known, the only completely reliable way to prevent rabies is to vaccinate the people at risk and check that their antibody response is adequate before they are exposed to infection.

A doctor who gave mouth-to-mouth respiration to an unsuspected case of rabies in Britain survived this extreme exposure. But the post-exposure prophylactic treatment available today cannot be relied upon to provide complete protection of medical staff against such a fatal disease (see page 110). These facts argue for a designated centre in

Britain for the care of patients suspected of having rabies. The staff of this centre would be fully vaccinated and could look after rabid patients without fear of infection.

People at risk from rabies

Unless rabies is reintroduced into Britain the only people at risk in this country are those who come into contact with imported animals at ports and in quarantine areas, those who work with exotic animals in zoos or laboratories, those who handle the virus itself in the manufacture of vaccines and for research, and close contacts of imported human cases. In areas of the world where rabies is endemic veterinary surgeons or other animal handlers, zoologists, and cave explorers are particularly likely to be exposed to infection.

For reasons which are unknown rabies is up to seven times commoner in men than in women: this also applies to animals. About half the cases of rabies are in children less than fifteen years old.

Incubation period

The interval between the bite, which introduces the virus through the skin, and the appearance of symptoms of rabies, indicating invasion of the central nervous system, is known as the incubation period. In rabies it is more variable than in any other disease, ranging from nine days to (reputedly) many years. In about 85 per cent of cases it lasts between two weeks and two months, but it tends to be longer after bites on the limbs (average fifty-two days) than after those on the face (average thirty-five days), and to be shorter in children. During this interval the virus probably lingers and multiplies in muscle cells at the site of the bite and then ascends inside the nerves to reach the brain and spinal cord.

Some of the very long incubation periods were probably explained by a second, more recent but perhaps less dramatic, exposure, which the patient had forgotten. Another explanation could be that the virus lies dormant somewhere in the nervous system until it is reactivated by another virus infection or some other kind of stress. Viruses of the herpes group behave in this way. After a childhood infection with chicken pox the virus lingers for many years in nerve ganglia, which are junction boxes just before the nerve enters the brain or spinal cord, but can be reactivated by some local mechanical irritant to cause herpes zoster or 'shingles'. Cold sores of the lips are caused by reactivation of herpes simplex virus which also hangs around in the nervous system. A new infection such as 'common cold' reawakens the virus. Human cases of rabies have been associated with rhinovirus ('common cold') and herpes simplex infections, and, in experimental animals, rabies encephalitis can be precipitated by stress or by injection of corticosteroid hormones which are normally produced by the adrenal cortex during stress.

36

Rabies in man

For those patients who suspect or know they have been bitten by a rabid animal the long and variable incubation period is a desperately worrying time. They feel as though a death sentence were hanging over them. No wonder that, amongst less resilient personalities, extreme anxiety may lead to symptoms of hysterical pseudorabies. In countries where rabies is endemic the mental anguish resulting from possible exposure to infection cannot be measured in such simple terms as the incidence of the disease or the numbers of people vaccinated.

Prelude to the disease ('prodromal symptoms')

The first sign that treatment has failed to prevent rabies virus invading the central nervous system is often a vague feverish illness. The patient feels generally unwell with loss of appetite, headache and other aches and pains, weakness, tiredness, and fever. The symptoms may resemble influenza, a common cold, or a sore throat. Rarely there are more severe symptoms of a chest infection including cough. The patient may feel nauseated and retch, vomit, or have stomach ache and diarrhoea. Patients who know that they have been exposed to rabies will naturally become anxious and apprehensive when they fall ill a few weeks or months after the bite, but a change in mood is often noticeable as an early symptom even in those who have not appreciated the threat of rabies. Restlessness, depression, a feeling of tension, a sense of foreboding, nightmares or inability to sleep, and lack of concentration have all been described.

None of these features is diagnostic or even particularly suggestive of rabies. The majority of patients develop a symptom which is, however, highly suggestive of impending rabies. They feel an abnormal sensation radiating from the site of the bite wound, which by now will have healed. Numbness, tingling ('pins and needles'), itching, coldness, burning, stabbing pain, or aching may be experienced in association with trembling or weakness of the affected limb. These prodromal symptoms, which are the prelude to the illness proper, last for a few hours to a few days.

At this stage, doctors who see the patient may well be baffled unless the past incident of animal bite is mentioned, or the healed bite wounds are noticed. Pain or abnormal sensation in the region of a wound scar should always prompt questions about possible animal bites, especially if the patient has been to a part of the world where rabies is still endemic, or if his occupation puts him at special risk. If the true diagnosis is not suspected the patient may be referred to inappropriate specialists such as ear, nose, and throat surgeons, or psychiatrists.

In man and in animals rabies can take two clincial forms. Both are the result of acute inflammation of the central nervous system. In the more familiar type, furious or agitated rabies, the brain itself is predominantly affected, whereas in the rarer paralytic or dumb form it is the spinal cord which is chiefly involved.

Furious rabies

If life is not prolonged by intensive care (see below) the average patient with furious rabies experiences a few days of horrifyingly hectic symptoms, including hydrophobia, interrupted by intervals of almost normal consciousness and comprehension, ending in coma, complete paralysis, and death within a week.

In order to understand the signs and symptoms of furious rabies it is necessary to know which parts of the brain are most severely inflamed. These include the brain stem, limbic system, and hypothalamus. The brain stem contains centres for the control of breathing (respiratory centre), for control of the calibre of blood vessels and activity of the heart (vasomotor centre), and for the sensation and muscular contraction in the tongue and throat (sensory and motor nuclei of IX, X, and XII cranial nerves). The circuits responsible for emotion, aggression, arousal, and sexuality are contained in the limbic system, amygdaloid nuclei, hippocampus, reticular-formation, and hypothalamus. The hypothalamus is also involved in temperature control, autonomic. nervous system activities (sweating, lacrimation, salivation etc.), and, through its protuberance, the pituitary gland, with control of the concentration of urine excreted by the kidneys.

Hydrophobia

Derived from two Greek words (ὕδωρ, φόβος), hydrophobia means 'dread of water' and was once used as an alternative name for rabies. Now, it refers to the most terrible and mysterious symptom in the whole of medicine. The patient picks up a cup to drink, but, even before the liquid has touched his lips, his arm shakes, and his body is contorted by violent jerky spasms of the diaphragm and other inspiratory muscles. The head is jerked back, the arms are thrown upwards and the spasm may affect other muscles until the whole body is arched backwards into an involuntary 'back-bend' (opisthotonos). At the same moment the patient experiences extreme terror. Hydrophobia may develop after initial difficulty in swallowing liquids or a feeling of tightness in the throat. Attempts to swallow may be defeated by spluttering and coughing as the liquid is inhaled into the windpipe and forced back through the nose. These episodes are frightening and uncomfortable in themselves and may help to build up or reinforce a fear of water. But sometimes the first attack of hydrophobia comes on dramatically, without any preceding difficulties with swallowing, and with no opportunity for establishing a conditioned reflex.

Some patients feel agonizing pain and constriction in the throat and larynx which makes them clutch at their throats. For many years this was thought to explain the terror of hydrophobia, but some patients with hydrophobia have specifically denied any pain in the throat.

The same combination of muscle spasm and terror can be triggered off by other stimuli such as a draught of air on the face. In this case the response is known as aerophobia (literally, 'dread of air'). This symptom is particularly common among South American patients, who frequently arrive at hospital swathed in heavy clothing to avoid exposure to draughts. Other potent stimuli include touching the back of the throat or the inside of the windpipe, splashing water on the skin, attempts to speak, loud noises, and bright lights. Hydrophobia may be produced by the sight, sound, or mention of water, or even by the arrival of someone whom the patient suspects may be bringing water. Patients may continue to eat solid food even though liquids induce hydrophobia. The patient with weakened swallowing muscles finds it easier to control a solid bolus of food than liquid which can slip down 'the wrong way' into the windpipe.

Patients show an extraordinary ambivalence about drinking. They avoid drinking for some time, fearing the effects, but finally become unbearably thirsty. Attempts to lift the cup to their lips are thwarted by violent trembling of the arm. They try desperately to snatch a sip of water before a last-minute terror makes them fling away the cup and dive under the bedclothes. During spasms the drink or saliva may be spat or coughed out in showers over bystanders. Patients may retch or vomit so violently that tears are made in the gullet near its junction with the stomach. Cries of alarm may be distorted by paralysis or swelling of the vocal cords which alter the voice so that shouts sound more like barks.

Spasms of hydrophobia tend to increase in frequency and intensity so that after a time they may happen spontaneously, without provocation by water or other stimuli, as though there were some irritant pacemaker within the brain. At the peak of an attack the whole nervous system seems to be aroused. The patient is in a state of extreme agitation and has frightening hallucinations. His face is a mask of terror. His body is racked with tremors or spasms. He may struggle frantically to free himself and try to escape from the room. Rarely he may attack and bite his attendants, an event which has been exaggerated in popular accounts of rabies. Breathing may stop because of continuous spasms of the breathing muscles, because the patient is choked by spasms of the throat or larynx, or because the respiratory centre in the brain stem ceases to function. The heart races but may suddenly stop beating because of stimulation of its inhibitor (vagus) nerves or because breathing has stopped and the blood is no longer oxygenated. Generalized convulsions, like epileptic fits, are the final event before death in at least a third of the cases.

In between these episodes of excitement, which last a few minutes, the patient may become clear-headed and calm, able to discuss the symptoms and to appreciate the nature of the disease. This is one of the most distressing features of rabies for the patient and for his attendants. Unless the patient is effectively drugged with analgesics, sedatives, or tranquillizers the suffering may have to be endured for several days until relieved at last by unconsciousness.

The mechanism of hydrophobia

It is difficult to fit all the reported facts about hydrophobia into one hypothetical mechanism, but here is an attempt to do so. The airways to the lungs are protected by powerful reflexes such as coughing and sneezing. Nerve cells in the lining of the nose, throat, larynx, windpipe, and elsewhere are sensitive to irritants such as touch, noxious fumes, and dust. These irritable receptors can activate reflex nerve circuits causing contraction of muscles in the air tubes and the muscles which cause inspiration and expiration. The result is usually a sharp breath in, followed by a transient closing or narrowing of the airway, and finally an explosive breath out – the cough or sneeze – which carries with it the irritant foreign body. There are two related mechanisms, the immersion and aspiration reflexes. The aspiration reflex is normally present only in very young infants. When an area at the back of the nose (epipharynx) is touched there are reflex contractions of the diaphragm, and increased blood pressure. The immersion reflex causes powerful breaths and slowing of the heart when the face, or more of the body, is immersed in cold water. Sudden cooling of the skin by immersion in water can cause uncontrollable gasping which may lead to aspiration.

These reflexes are concerned with survival, protecting the airway from blockage by an inhaled foreign body. Infection of the brain with rabies virus might selectively destroy the inhibitory circuits which normally damp down these reflexes and keep them under control. Removal of the damping would allow a grossly exaggerated response to the stimuli which normally provoke the reflex. These stimuli include some of the ones which also cause hydrophobia. The major stimulus to hydrophobia is, of course, the attempt to drink water. In rabies the associated weakness of swallowing (pharyngeal) muscles in the throat allows water to come into contact with the entrance to the larynx and the back of the nose. This will stimulate coughing and those other reflexes which cause a preliminary, sharp, inspiratory breath and may explain the inspiratory muscle spasms of hydrophobia. The terror of rabies can only be explained by the inflammation of circuits concerned with arousing the whole system at times of danger or anger. These circuits are linked to those parts of the brain responsible for emotions including fear and aggression. The unique predilection which the rabies virus has for these particular areas of the brain stem and limbic system in man explains why hydrophobia is not seen in other brain infections, and is never seen in rabid animals. Only in rabies is there intense inflammation of these areas at a time when the patients' preserved consciousness makes them prey to the resulting emotional disturbances including terror.

Other features of furious rabies

Since the rabies virus can affect almost any part of the brain it is not surprising that a very wide range of symptoms and signs has been described. Despite the severity of the brain-stem encephalitis there may be no abnormal signs when the patient's nervous system is examined in the conventional way. But if such a patient is asked to swallow the saliva accumulated in his mouth, or if a window is opened so that a draught blows on his face a typical hydrophobic spasm may announce the diagnosis.

Neck stiffness, suggesting inflammation of the membranes covering the brain (meningitis), is quite unusual in rabies, and the cerebrospinal fluid obtained by lumbar puncture is completely normal in up to three quarters of the cases.

A staring appearance, the eyes wide open and the pupils dilated, is said to be characteristic of rabies. The cranial nerves, which arise directly from the brain, may be affected causing paralysis of the eye muscles producing a squint or drooping of the eyelids, or paralysis of one side of the face, the throat, tongue, or vocal cords. Signs of stimulation of the autonomic nervous system, perhaps at the level of the hypothalamus, include increased salivation so that frothy secretions dribble from the gaping mouth, excessive lacrimation (watering of the eyes), sweating, and goose flesh. There is usually a fever which may be so high (more than 42°C) that the brain is damaged. In some patients the temperature-regulating mechanism in the brain is destroyed, so that body temperature may swing above and below normal. Erratic secretion of antidiuretic hormone by the posterior part of the pituitary gland may cause fluctuations in the volume and concentration of urine. In a small minority of patients there are bizarre abnormalities of function of the hypothalamus and amygdaloid nuclei producing increased libido (satyriasis, nymphomania), which drove one patient to attempt sexual intercourse thirty times in one day. Patients may also experience severe pain in the penis, unprovoked penile erection (priapism), and spontaneous ejaculation of semen, and may commit acts of indecent exposure and attempted rape.

Outside the central nervous system rabies virus has been isolated from almost every tissue and organ examined. It is distributed via the network of nerves and in rare instances through the blood stream. Infection of the salivary and lacrimal glands is important in man because it creates the risk of transmission to another human being (see above). The effects of rabies virus on the functioning of organs outside the nervous system are unknown. Inflammation of the heart muscle (myocarditis) has been found in some patients who died from rabies. The virus was isolated from the heart in a proportion of these cases and many of them had signs of disturbed function of the heart before they died. Irregular heart rhythm, heart rates that were too rapid or too slow, and other electrical abnormalities were often detected by the electrocardiogram, and a few patients showed a fall in blood pressure and even heart failure. The pneumonia which usually develops in those patients who survive more than a few days may be due to rabies virus or to a bacterial infection.

When patients with furious rabies lapse into coma they become virtually indistinguishable from people suffering from other virus infections of the brain. Periods of excitement and jerky breathing may still occur from time to time but this type of irregular breathing, known as Biot's or cluster breathing, is seen in other brain infections. Generalized paralysis eventually ensues. The ones who are not supported by intensive care usually die on the second to fourth day of their illness and very rarely survive longer than a week.

The course of the disease is best illustrated by an account of an actual case. A 29-year-old Nigerian, who was a rural health inspector for the sleeping sickness survey on the Jos Plateau, was riding his motor bike when a dog ran up barking and nipped at his right ankle. He went to a local dispensary where the two small wounds were cleaned with iodine. There was nothing remarkable about the dog's appearance and, since dogs often chase bicycles, the possibility of rabies was dismissed. The dog had run off after the incident and so could not be examined.

The bite wounds healed up, but 36 days after the attack the patient noticed pain and numbness around the scars of the bite wounds. These feelings continued and three days later he developed fever with headache. Suspecting malaria, which is very common in Nigeria, he decided to treat himself with chloroquine. He put the tablets on his tongue and took a sip of water to help swallow them. As the water entered his mouth, 'all hell was let loose'. There was a violent involuntary gasp and he choked. The pills shot out of his mouth and water came back down his nose and was inhaled into his windpipe. Far worse, there was an inexplicable and overwhelming feeling of terror, 'I felt that I wanted to run through the window, to get away'. He could not understand this reaction. Although he had learned about rabies as part of his medical training he still did not associate his symptoms with this disease. So vivid and frightening was the experience that he dared not eat or drink for the next two days, 'I knew that the terror would return'. But eventually he managed to swallow some dry bread. He was admitted to a mission hospital where he was given intravenous fluids because he could not drink. He was then transferred 200 miles by road to Ahmadu Bello University Hospital in Zaria.

When first examined in Zaria he was found to be an alert, intelligent man who spoke English fluently. Apart from loss of feeling on the back of his throat and around the bite wound there seemed to be nothing wrong. But when he was asked to swallow, or was exposed to a draught by opening a window, he was shaken by jerky spasms of inspiratory muscles and looked terrified, cowering beneath the bedclothes. These attacks felt like 'electric shocks' and caused 'confusion of the brain'. He absolutely denied any pain in the throat but feared that drinking water might block his breathing.

Intensive care was not feasible, but this unfortunate man was made as comfortable as possible with tranquillizing and pain-killing drugs. Calm reassurance persuaded him to swallow porridge and even water. He slept peacefully after being given the drugs, but always awoke frightened, confused, and hallucinated.

During the next thirty-six hours he became increasingly excitable, and required frequent doses of the drugs. At times he was confused and wild, knocking over the bedside table and shouting that he was dying. Then he sank back into coma. His breathing was irregular with pauses of several minutes between groups of breaths. He sweated profusely and tears ran continuously from his eyes. By this time drugs were no longer necessary and had been stopped, but he remained comatose and unresponsive with generally floppy muscles. He died peacefully seven days after the first symptoms.

Rabies virus was isolated from his brain after death, but the diagnosis had already been confirmed while he was alive by examining a small piece of skin by the fluorescent antibody technique.

Paralytic or dumb rabies

Rabies takes this form in less than a fifth of all cases. Paralytic rabies can follow bites by dogs but is most likely to occur in those bitten by rabid bats, and in those who have been given rabies vaccine. The different pattern of nervous system disease may be explained by a slight alteration in the properties of the virus resulting from its passage through the bat, or to modification of its mode of attack by the host's response to the vaccine.

The most famous outbreak of paralytic rabies was in Trinidad. During the years 1929-31 a mysterious and invariably fatal disease appeared there. Twenty people, most of them children, were affected. The illness usually started with fever and headache. Soon there was burning, tingling, numbness, cramp, or weakness in one foot, followed by a gradually ascending paralysis and loss of feeling. The legs, trunk, arms, and finally the muscles of breathing and swallowing were affected in turn. Constipation and inability to empty the bladder, high fever, and profuse sweating were also noticed. The patients were at first fully conscious and rational, but finally became delirious and comatose. Some developed a stiff neck, suggesting meningitis, and some dribbled saliva because they were unable to swallow it. Terminal hydrophobic spasms were seen in only one case.

The patients seen at the beginning of this strange epidemic did not remember being bitten. Later a woman who had been woken by pain found that her toe was bleeding. A bat flew from the foot of her bed! Four weeks later she noticed numbness and paralysis spreading from the bitten foot: this ultimately involved muscles of respiration. She died after a week's illness.

At first this epidemic was attributed to an unusually severe form of paralytic poliomyelitis, or to botulism, caused by food poisoning by *Clostridium botulinum* bacteria. The true cause was finally established by isolating rabies virus from human victims, local vampire bats (*Desmodus rotundus*), and from farm animals which had also been dying of a strange paralytic illness. The human victims must have been bitten by rabid vampire bats while they were asleep. Most of them had not noticed the wounds.

In paralytic rabies it is the spinal cord and the lowest part of the brain stem (medulla oblongata) which bears the brunt of the inflammation. Equally affected are those parts of the spinal cord which transmit muscle-activating (motor) impulses from the brain, and the parts relaying sensory signals about touch and temperature from the skin. Inflammatory changes are also found in the nerves which sprout from the spinal cord.

Most patients with paralytic rabies do not experience hydrophobia at any stage of their illness, but in a few it may be represented by some terminal spasms of the throat. The course of the disease is less stormy than in furious rabies. Even without intensive care patients may survive for up to 30 days before they succumb to paralysis of the breathing and swallowing muscles, as do patients with paralytic poliomyelitis.

Clinical diagnosis of human rabies

Rabies should be suspected in any patient who develops severe neurological symptoms after being bitten by an animal. Sometimes, however, the bite is forgotten, the doctor forgets to ask about bites, or the patient arrives in hospital unconscious with no helpful relative to tell the story. Many medical textbooks state that furious rabies is easily diagnosed clinically, i.e. by examining the patient. Yet patients are sometimes misdiagnosed. Their altered mood, hallucinations, and bizarre behaviour raises suspicions of psychiatric disease or malingering and they may end up in a mental institution.

Since rabies is such a dreaded and notorious disease it is not surprising that some hysterical people should imagine that they are suffering from it. These patients imitate what they know or imagine to be the features of rabies, concentrating on its more spectacular manifestations, such as aggression, biting, barking, and hydrophobia. Their displays are exaggerated caricatures of hydrophobia which do not reproduce accurately its true features. The absence of fever, objective neurological signs, and abnormal laboratory results, the patients' failure to deteriorate and their eventual 'recovery' all point to a diagnosis of hysterical pseudorabies (also called rabies hysteria, lyssaphobia, and hydrophobia-phobia). The interval between bite and appearance of symptoms in these cases may be only a few days, impossibly short for rabies incubation. Knowledge of a patient's previous personality may help in the assessment.

The muscle spasms of furious rabies may suggest tetanus, a disease resulting from the effect on the central nervous system of a potent toxin from *Clostridium tetani* bacteria. Tetanus may follow an animal bite or other dirty wound. Its incubation period is usually shorter than that of rabies, at less than two weeks, but rarely may exceed three months. A prominent symptom of tetanus is inability to open the mouth, due to rigidity of the chewing muscles (masseters). This symptom, known as trismus, gives rise to the popular name 'lockjaw'. Certain groups of muscles, especially those of the face, back, and abdomen, go into a state of sustained contraction. This does not happen in rabies. Superimposed are occasional spasms brought on by stimuli such as touch, pain, noise, and light. Although true hydrophobia is not seen in tetanus patients, they may have painful spasms when they attempt to swallow. Severe spasms of the larynx or the breathing muscles can cause asphyxiation and fits. There are disturbances of the autonomic nervous system such as excessive sweating, a very rapid heart rate, and fluctuations in blood pressure. Loss of body temperature control is another feature. Tetanus, unlike rabies, does not cause inflammation of the brain, but complications such as asphyxiation or high fever may damage the brain. In tetanus the cerebrospinal fluid is said to be invariably normal, whereas in at least a quarter of rabies cases it contains increased numbers of cells (lymphocytes) and increased amounts of protein as in other brain inflammations caused by viruses. The severity of tetanus varies. At one extreme there is mild stiffness of a single limb, at the other there are frequent generalized spasms and a very high mortality in untreated patients. Effective modern treatment

David A. Warrell

for severe tetanus includes making the patient sleepy with sedative drugs, preventing spasms by paralysing the muscles with curare (a drug derived from a South American arrow poison), ventilating the lungs artificially with a machine through a tube inserted into the windpipe, and preventing complications such as chest infections, bed sores, high temperatures, and autonomic nervous-system complications. If the patient can be kept alive by these means until the effect of the toxin on the brain has worn off, complete recovery is possible. Since there is no encephalitis, there need be no permanent brain damage.

Thus tetanus and rabies, although superficially similar in their effects on the body, cause very different disturbances in the nervous system and have a different prognosis for recovery.

Other virus infections of the brain (encephalitides) can cause fever, headache, psychological changes, agitated behaviour, signs of nervous system damage, coma, and convulsion. But hydrophobia does not occur and there are rarely signs of intense brain-stem inflammation in a conscious patient. World-wide, an enormous range of viruses, many of them transmitted by insects and ticks (Arboviruses, Togaviruses), can cause encephalitis. In Britain, herpes simplex, measles, mumps, and herpes zoster infections may be associated with encephalitis. A special risk after monkey bites is Herpes simiae (B virus) (see below).

Many other microorganisms can infect the brain. Two most important tropical infections which may be seen in Britain in patients who have been abroad are cerebral malaria and typhoid fever. Confusion, irritability, and loss of consciousness may be prominent clinical features in both diseases. The important point is that, unlike rabies, these treatable infections are easily diagnosed (by microscopical examination of the blood in malaria, and by incubating the blood to grow the bacteria in typhoid). These possibilities must not be overlooked in favour of a virus encephalitis when travellers from overseas develop signs of cerebral disease.

Delirium tremens ('the shakes' or 'D.T.s') is a dramatic illness seen in severe alcoholics who are in a state of alcoholic withdrawal. They have frightening hallucinations, such as seeing unnaturally-coloured wild animals. They tremble all over and become confused, agitated, or even maniacal. They may have difficulty swallowing and may develop a high fever and convulsions. These features could suggest a diagnosis of furious rabies: one reported case of recovery from rabies in the USA in 1913 was probably suffering from delirium tremens. Victor Babès, director of the Bucharest Institute of Pathology and Bacteriology at the beginning of this century and author of an outstanding textbook on rabies, mentioned this condition as a differential diagnosis of rabies. He pointed out that delirium and hallucinations are early symptoms in alcoholic delirium tremens, whereas they develop later in the clinical course of rabies. Some types of strokes and epileptic fits may mimic rabies, but there will be no association with animal bites and no hydrophobia.

Finally, various poisons, drugs, and plant toxins can produce spasms, agitation, hallucinations, psychiatric disturbances, signs of autonomic nervous system stimulation, and convulsions. These features could cause confusion with rabies. The compounds include strychnine, phenothiazines, tryparsamide, atropine-like compounds, and cannabis. Only a good clinical history can sort out these problems.

An ascending paralysis, similar to the paralytic form of rabies, can happen as a complication of the older types of rabies vaccines (see page 105). It is difficult to put a figure to the incidence of post-vaccinal reactions. The most that can be safely said is that the more diligently they are sought the higher the incidence. The mildest type of reaction is a nerve inflammation or neuritis affecting either nerves arising from the brain (cranial nerves VII, III, IX or X) or those arising from the spinal cord (radial, ulnar, or sciatic nerves). A more severe form causes paralysis and loss of sensation of both legs with disturbance of the control of bladder and bowels. Complete recovery within a few weeks is the rule in these types of reaction. The most severe illness starts with fever, headache, severe backache, and restlessness. During the next few days paralysis and numbness spread upwards from the legs to the face. A third of these patients will die. The overall mortality from post-vaccinal reactions is about 15 per cent. Reactions are exceptionally common (up to 1 in 230 courses of vaccine) and severe amongst the Japanese who seem to be uniquely susceptible to a delayed cerebral type of reaction which produces psychiatric symptoms.

Post-vaccinal reactions are distinguished from rabies by their earlier onset, usually within two weeks of the first dose of vaccine, while the course of injections is still in progress. Unlike rabies victims most cases recover rapidly. Laboratory tests to detect an underlying immunological defect may help to distinguish these reactions from rabies.

Paralytic poliomyelitis has been confused with paralytic rabies, as in the Trinidad epidemic described above. Poliomyelitis may be suspected in the presence of an epidemic. Apart from its lower mortality it may be distinguished from rabies by the absence of numbness or other sensory disturbances. In poliomyelitis, fever will have subsided by the time paralysis develops, whereas in rabies it is at its height at that time. The cells in the cerebrospinal fluid may be different in the two diseases and ultimately poliomyelitis virus may be isolated from the cerebrospinal fluid, throat, or stools.

Various other diseases which cause an ascending paralysis such as acute infectious polyneuritis and syphilis of the spinal cord may have to be distinguished from rabies by appropriate examinations of the cerebrospinal fluid and blood.

David A. Warrell

Monkeys are almost as dangerous as dogs to human health. A patient who develops severe neurological symptoms after a bite or other close contact with a Rhesus monkey (*Macaca mulatta*) or other asiatic macaque could be suffering from *Herpes simiae* (B virus) encephalomyelitis. At least 20 human cases have now been reported, all but two of them fatal. Blisters may be found in the monkey's mouth and appear around the patient's wound a few days after the bite. An influenza-like illness develops 3 to 24 days later. There is neck stiffness, difficulty in swallowing, numbness, and ascending paralysis. Death is caused by paralysis of breathing and swallowing muscles. The diagnosis is confirmed by virus isolation and blood tests. A large number of monkeys is imported for medical research, vaccine production, etc. and so there is a real risk of simian herpes infections in the people who have to handle them.

Prevention of human rabies

Attempts to prevent rabies are likely to be far more successful than attempts to cure it. If the risk of rabies in certain places, situations, and occupations (e.g. cave exploring, animal collecting, veterinary work) is appreciated, pre-exposure vaccination can provide excellent protection. In areas where rabies is endemic all unnecessary contact with domestic and wild animals should be avoided. Wild animals that seem attractively docile should not be touched, for rabies might well be the cause of their apparent tameness.

Animal bites anywhere in the world should be taken seriously because of the risk of any infection, not only rabies. Wounds should be washed vigorously with soap and water, making sure that any dirt is removed. In countries where rabies exists grazes and scratches which might have been contaminated by an animal's saliva should also be cleaned carefully. After rinsing away the soap with clean water the ideal treatment is to apply a 0·1 per cent solution of centrimide ('Savlon', 'Cetavlon') or some other quaternary ammonium compound which will kill rabies virus. Wounds should not be stitched or covered with dressings. Advice from a local doctor should be sought and, if there is rabies in that locality, some attempt should be made to get the biting animal caught and examined by a veterinarian. Decisions about post-exposure treatment with vaccine and antiserum must be made as soon as possible. People who are bitten by animals while they are abroad often do not approach a doctor until they get back to this country, perhaps weeks later. It is then too late for effective treatment and immunization, and it will be almost impossible to get any information about the biting animal.

Rabies in man

Risks of immunization versus risks of developing rabies: the doctor's dilemma

In parts of the world where rabies is endemic doctors are frequently faced with the problem of treating patients who have been bitten by animals. The wound should always be cleaned as described above and the risk of tetanus considered, but rabies vaccine and antiserum cannot be used indiscriminately because of the risk of severe reactions. Patients with severe and multiple bites especially involving the face, those bitten by animals showing obvious signs of rabies, and those bitten by any wild animal should be given full immunization without hesitation. Confirmation of rabies in the biting animal is valuable if it can be achieved rapidly, by fluorescent methods. But delay can be dangerous. Recently in the USA a woman who had been bitten by a bat was started on the full recommended programme of immunization 44 hours later, after the bat had been proved to have rabies. In this case the delay was fatal for she developed rabies after 25 days. Usually, treatment must be started before any laboratory results are known. In the developing countries where rabies is most common there is the added problem of expense, supply, and preservation of vaccines and antiserum. In these countries dog-bite victims have to be selected for antirabies treatment on the basis of information about the circumstances of the bite (e.g. whether or not it was provoked) and the behaviour and appearance of the animal.

In the privileged western countries, the availability of newer, safer, and more potent vaccines, such as human diploid cell strain vaccine, the use of human antirabies globulin rather than equine rabies antiserum, and the relative rarity of rabies have combined to virtually eliminate this medical dilemma.

Management of human rabies

In the past patients with rabies have been subjected to all manner of painful, barbaric, and useless remedies. In Britain, even until the beginning of the last century, rabies victims might be smothered or bled to death by their well-meaning friends and relations. More merciful forms of euthanasia have also been advocated. In many African countries these patients are sent away from hospital to die at home with their families. This practice ignores their suffering and exposes the relatives to the risk of infection.

Until recently rabies was regarded by most experts as an inevitably fatal disease. More than a dozen reports of alleged human recoveries from rabies had appeared before 1970, but in none was the diagnosis proven. Severe tetanus, which has features in common with rabies, can be successfully managed by sedation, curarization, mechanical ventilation, and energetic supportive and nursing care. It seemed logical to try this same regime in rabies. In 1956 the life of a 65-year-old rabies patient in El Kettar Hospital in Algeria was prolonged until the eleventh day of his illness using this treatment. Results were less impressive in sixteen other patients subsequently treated in the same way. Patients usually died with failure of the heart and circulation about five days after the start of their illness. During the next fifteen years evidence of severe disorders of the heart, lungs, and metabolism was discovered in rabies victims which helped to explain these deaths. Surprisingly, the brain damage in rabies patients appeared no more severe than in some other virus infections of the brain (e.g. herpes simplex encephalitis) from which patients could recover.

Amongst a group of rabies experts working with the Center for Disease Control in Atlanta, Georgia, USA, there grew a new enthusiasm for the use of intensive care in rabies. They believed that, given time, the encephalitis might resolve by natural processes if only the patient could be kept alive by preventing dangerous complications. This radical or 'aggressive' approach to treatment demanded the full resources of modern medical technology. Continuous monitoring of the heart's electrical activity (electrocardiogram) and other vital measures of bodily function were needed to give early warning of complications. Mechanical ventilation of the lungs, and artificial regulation of the heart beat by an electrical stimulator (cardiac pacemaker) were used to support failing systems. Biochemical disturbances, excessive brain swelling, epileptic fits and infections were treated with drugs and the nursing care was meticulous. Soon the lives of three proven cases of rabies had been prolonged by these means to 28, 64, and 133 days after the start of symptoms. The stage was set for a dramatic success.

Recovery from rabies?

In 1970, six-year-old Matthew Winkler was bitten on the left thumb by a rabid Big Brown bat (*Eptesicus fuscus*) in Ohio, USA. When the diagnosis of rabies in the bat had been confirmed four days later a course of vaccine was started, but no rabies antiserum or human anti-rabies globulin was given. Twenty days after the bite and two days after finishing the two week course of vaccination, the boy noticed pain in the neck and in the next few days he became feverish and dizzy, lost his appetite and began to vomit. Because there was no improvement by the fifth day of his illness, despite antibiotic treatment, he was admitted to hospital. He developed pains all over, he seemed listless, and his neck became stiff. By the fifteenth day of the illness his condition had deteriorated. Abnormalities of the nervous system were obvious. His behaviour was odd, he stopped speaking, showed signs of a stroke affecting the left side of his body, and finally went unconscious. A small piece of his brain was removed to help diagnosis, but microscopical examination only showed inflammation (encephalitis) and did not prove rabies. His heart began to beat irregularly, there were problems with his breathing, the pressure inside his skull rose because of brain swelling, and he began to have fits. A tube was inserted into his windpipe to improve breathing. His fits were treated with an anticonvulsant drug.

A turning point was reached after he had been unconscious for nine days. There were signs of improvement, and during the next few months he made a complete recovery with no residual damage to his nervous system. Matthew Winkler was very thoroughly investigated. The diagnosis of rabies, as opposed to post-vaccinal encephalitis (see above), was based on finding concentrations of rabies antibodies in his blood and cerebrosphinal fluid which were considered too high to be explained by his course of antirabies vaccine. The clinical features were, however, more reminiscent of post-vaccinal encephalitis and some doubt may remain about the true diagnosis of this most important and fascinating case.

The report of Matthew Winkler's illness was particularly valuable in inspiring a complete revision of doctors' attitudes to the outlook and management of rabies patients. In 1972 a 45-year-old woman also survived a severe illness which had started 21 days after she was bitten by her dog. This happened in an area of Argentina where rabies is endemic. Again the diagnosis was made from the blood and cerebrospinal fluid antibody levels and, since she had been given vaccine, the illness could have been a severe post vaccinal encephalomyelitis. Unlike Matthew Winkler this patient had a long illness, but had virtually recovered after 13 months.

Unfortunately, subsequent attempts to cure rabies with intensive care have failed in USA, Brazil, India, and England. These experiences suggest that, after all, it is the severity of the brain inflammation which poses the greatest barrier to survival. Yet intensive care remains the only known method of prolonging the lives of rabies patients.

Many different types of treatment have been tried but none has proved effective in the slightest degree. The use of vaccine for active immunization is obviously pointless once the disease is rampant in the central nervous system. Treatment with ready-made antibodies in the form of equine antiserum or human antirabies globulin does, however, seem logical for the virus is widely disseminated throughout the body.

The few antiviral agents which are available have some effect on rabies virus in the test tube but are useless in living animals or human patients. This is hardly surprising, for these compounds are structurally related to parts of the DNA molecule and therefore most likely to be effective against viruses which contain DNA. Rabies virus contains only RNA. Substances which have been shown experimentally to stimulate the body's own antiviral substance, interferon, are also ineffective.

Antibodies produced by the patient, although directed against rabies virus, may incidentally destroy those nerve cells containing the virus. Antibodies might thus prove more deadly than the virus itself. This interesting hypothesis prompted trials of treatment designed to suppress the immunological response to infection. Drugs such as methyl prednisolone were used and even exchange blood transfusion to eliminate circulating lytic antibody, but all to no avail.

Despite our increasing understanding of the disturbances of bodily function in rabies, and the promising results of intensive care, this disease remains the most terrible and hopeless of all human infections.

Prevention is the only answer to the problem of human rabies. Especially in the poorer developing countries, money should be used for prevention, including the emergency treatment of animal bites and immunization, rather than for attempts at intensive care. In many countries the only action which is practicable and humane once the disease has developed is to admit the patients to hospital, relieve their fear and pain by gentle attention and adequate doses of drugs, and prevent their transmitting the infection.

4

Rabies in animals

D. A. HAIG

Firm diagnosis of rabies was not possible until 1903 when the Italian scientist Negri showed that under the microscope he could demonstrate darkly staining bodies, unique to rabies, in certain nerve cells of the brains of rabid animals. Nevertheless the clinical signs of the disease seen in epizooties are usually so characteristic that diagnosis by trained observers is remarkably accurate. There are numerous graphic descriptions of disease dating back to Grecian times which cannot be mistaken for any other disease. However, isolated cases appearing in places where the disease is unknown or has long been absent are difficult to recognize and may be wrongly diagnosed as a bone stuck in the throat, the nervous form of canine distemper, or even road accidents.

Unless veterinary surgeons and indeed the majority of owners of animals are aware of the various forms the disease can assume and are constantly on the alert for such signs, the first cases in countries such as Britain could be missed and the disease could even become firmly established before its presence was recognized.

All warm-blooded animals, even birds, are susceptible to rabies. Tortoises and possibly all reptiles are less susceptible. The virus multiplies very slowly or not at all at the low body temperature of these animals and in mammals, such as bats, during hibernation.

In all warm-blooded animals the incubation period and the symptoms have marked basic similarities. The length of the incubation period depends mainly on the amount of virus that enters the body following bites or licking of abraded surfaces. However, other factors also have a marked influence. These are the site of the bite or abrasion, the treatment given to the wounds, the strain of virus, and possibly pregnancy and such indefinable factors as severe mental stress.

Some of the information on the length of the incubation period has been obtained in laboratory trials. These are comparatively sparse, not only because they require very special facilities but also because there is a natural reluctance on the part of laboratory workers to undertake some of the more horrific experiments, and such work is, today, difficult to justify. Therefore, we must rely to a large extent on observations made on naturally occurring cases, knowing that some of these clinical observations could be unreliable. The incubation periods shown in the table have been gathered from various sources and give some idea of the range that has been reported.

| | Incubation period of rabies | | |
	Minimum	Maximum	Usual
Dog	5 days	14 months	2−8 weeks
Cat	...	...	2−4 weeks
Cattle	10 days	1 year	3−4 weeks
Sheep	14 days	...	2−4 weeks
Horse	15 days	15 months	8−12 weeks
Pig	8 days	...	4 weeks
Deer	...	...	3 weeks
Fox	10 days	3−5 months	2−3 weeks

From these figures it is apparent that, while the incubation period is usually about 2 to 4 weeks, it can vary considerably. For reasons which will be discussed later it is the long-drawn-out periods which cause problems.

As discussed in Chapter 1, the virus of rabies enters nerve processes at the site of the infected wound or abrasion and travels along these nerves to the brain. The distance of the portal of entry from the brain can markedly affect the incubation period; bites in the face and neck are notoriously dangerous because so little time is available for preventive vaccination or the natural defence mechanisms of the body to be effective. Conversely, bites on the extremities such as the feet are usually followed by long incubation periods and sometimes the virus never reaches the brain. Not all the virus that enters the body enters nerve cells, and some stimulates the antibody-forming system with the result that in those cases with long incubation periods, and in some which fail to react after exposure, high levels of antibody are produced. The virus appears in the salivary glands soon after beginning to multiply in the brain. These glands become demonstrably infected with virus at about the same time as the appearance of brain symptoms in foxes or even shortly before in dogs.

The incubation period can also be affected depending on whether the site of entry is covered by fur, wool, or clothing which removes most of the saliva from the attacking animal's teeth. It has been reported that men who had been savagely attacked by rabid wolves seldom developed rabies when the bites were made through thick clothing. Similarly dogs and sheep may be protected by their fur or wool. Unfortunately, horses and cattle are highly inquisitive and cannot resist inspecting animals such as dogs, foxes, or even mongooses showing abnormal behaviour. They tend to resent intrusions into their territory. As a result when they are bitten it is usually in the lip or muzzle. The proportion of these animals which develop symptoms is usually high and the incubation period short. Infection following inhalation is possible but must be rare other than in areas heavily contaminated with virus, such as bat caves in America.

The strain of virus also affects the incubation period. Sir Christopher Andrewes, the doyen of British virology, has stressed the fact that even viruses have to struggle for existence in this competitive world. Like the dinosaur they must disappear unless they adapt to changing circumstances. The fact that rabies virus has survived over the centuries with all the accompanying changes of animal population and behaviour shows how adaptable it is. Rapid passage of any virus, for example, that of myxomatosis of rabbits, in a highly susceptible population 'hots up' the strain by the natural selection of highly virulent variants from the mixed population of virus present in an infected animal, because the most lethal forms have the quickest effect, and are therefore the first to be passed on. The incubation period of such highly virulent strains which flourish at the height of an epizooty is comparatively short; but when new victims are few and far between, because many have died or become immune, natural selection favours the less virulent variants.

The effect of vaccination on the incubation period of rabies is not known with any certainty. Vaccines are regularly used with the object of aborting the development of symptoms in human beings who have been bitten by rabid animals. Therefore it is possible that when the vaccine is given some time after exposure and fails to prevent entry of virus into the brain it could nonetheless have extended the incubation period.

After two cases of rabies in England in 1969 and 1970 in dogs which had spent the statutory six months in quarantine, the Waterhouse Committee recommended that all dogs entering quarantine in Britain should be vaccinated to minimize the risk of accidental infection in the kennels (which was thought to have happened to the Camberley dog, Fritz, in 1969). However, this procedure might be ill-advised as it could lead to a delay in the onset of symptoms beyond the quarantine period of six months in dogs exposed to infection before entering the country. Support for this supposition is provided by the observation published on the Newmarket case of rabies in which the disease appeared in a dog nine months after importation from Pakistan (three months after release from quarantine). This dog was said to have been vaccinated three times at intervals of about a year. There was no history of infection in other animals held in the quarantine kennel at the time.

Whether pregnancy has a delaying effect on the development of the disease is not known for certain but a case in which this possibility was suspected has been reported. Because the hormonal changes that take place during pregnancy may affect the course of diseases of the brain, this possibility should not be ignored.

In some cases, where there is an unusually long interval between attack by a presumed infected animal and the onset of symptoms, the attacking animal may well have been free from the disease and the infection may actually have been transmitted later, on some apparently trivial occasion. Although the onset of the symptoms of rabies is generally preceded by a clearly definable incubation period after exposure to the virus, the history of naturally occurring cases, no matter how conscientiously recorded and presented, may easily be at fault when all the circumstances cannot be known or verified.

It is also possible that in some animals rabies virus may persist in a dormant state. In most communicable diseases it is commonly observed that there are periods of high incidence followed by virtual disappearance of the disease. This is presumably because the virus has difficulty in finding susceptible hosts since most have either died of the infection or have developed immunity. The sudden unexplained reappearance of the disease, apparently from nowhere, might suggest spontaneous origin of virus. However, a more likely explanation is that the virus may occasionally persist in a dormant phase and be re-activated by severe emotional disturbance or similar stress. Well-known examples of such re-activation in man are herpes simplex infections (cold sores) in patients under immunosuppression following organ transplant. In cattle, fatal recurrences of diseases such as redwater may follow vaccination with mild attenuated virus vaccines or surgical removal of the spleen. It is thus feasible that in some animals which receive only small doses of low virulence rabies virus in some part of the body distant from the head, such as the tail or paw, the virus could remain dormant and be activated at some time later by severe stress.

Rabies is a disease of the central nervous system. Thus the clinical signs are behavioural and relate to damage of the brain and spinal cord. The disease may be divided roughly into three phases: early, excitative, and paralytic. The phases usually overlap and the first two may be absent or inapparent. When the period of excitation predominates, the disease is commonly known as 'furious' rabies; the term 'dumb' rabies is used when paralysis is the main symptom. It is extremely rare for animals that have developed nervous symptoms to recover from the disease.

Dogs

Dogs, and to a lesser extent cats, are considered most likely to be the vehicles by which rabies would enter an isolated country such as

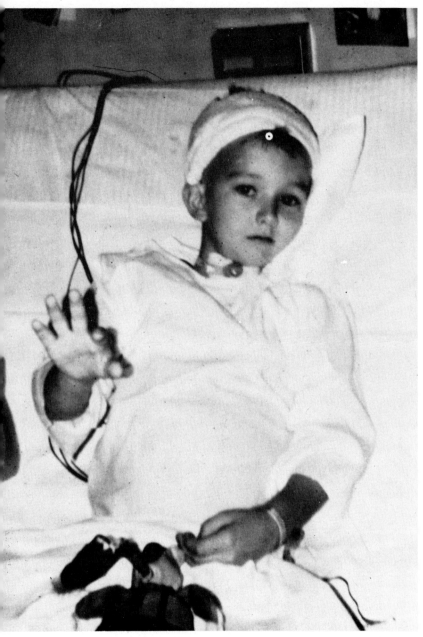

1. A survivor? Matthew Winkler appeared to contract rabies at the age of six after being bitten by a bat. After intensive care he survived and is shown here during his convalescense. (*Photograph provided by Dr Michael Hattwick*)

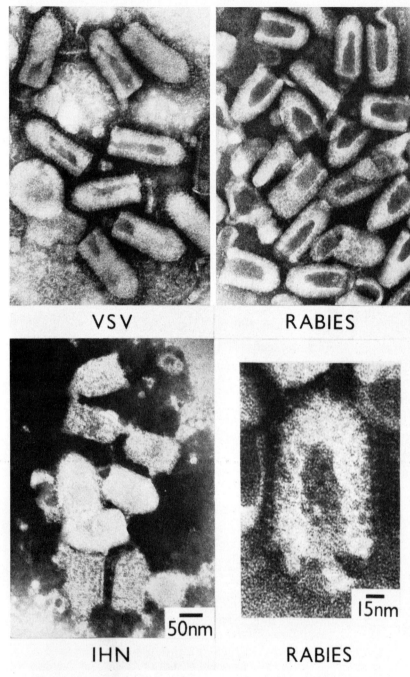

2. Electron micrographs of vesicular stomatitis, rabies, and infectious haematopoietic necrosis viruses. The electron micrograph of rabies virus at the higher magnification shows the spike projections and honeycomb structure described in Chapter 2. (*Photograph by C.J. Smale*)

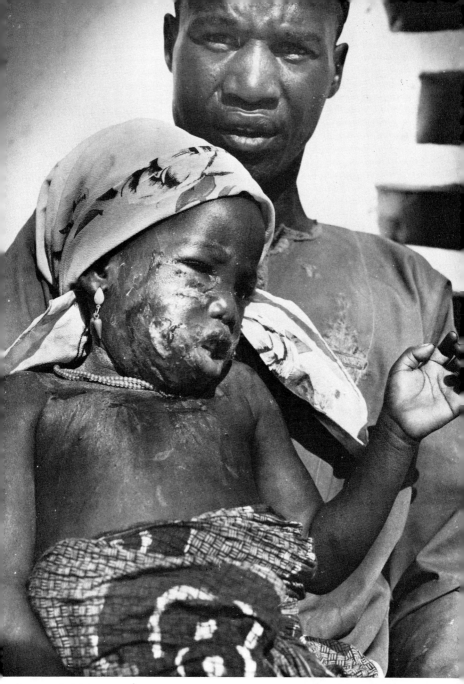

3. Severe facial bite wounds caused by a rabid dog. The patient, a five-year-old Nigerian girl, arrived at hospital 15 hours after being bitten. The wounds were cleaned with cetrimide solution. She was given rabies antiserum and a three-week course of daily injections of anti-rabies vaccine followed by booster doses 10 and 20 days later. Rabies was successfully prevented in this case. (*Photograph by Dr D.A. Warrell*)

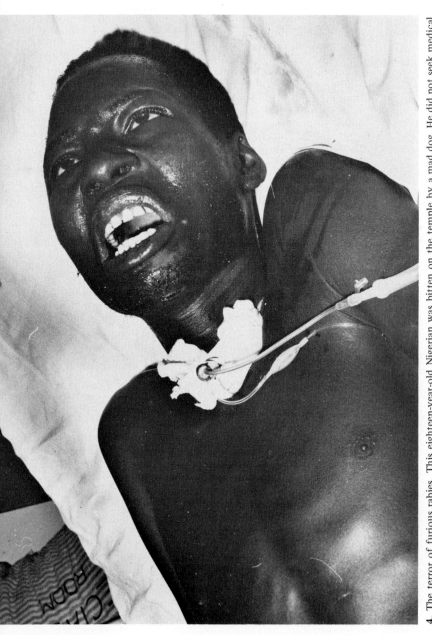

4. The terror of furious rabies. This eighteen-year-old Nigerian was bitten on the temple by a mad dog. He did not seek medical treatment until, only 13 days later, he developed classical hydrophobia. In hospital, a tube was inserted into the windpipe (tracheostomy) to prevent his asphyxiating during the hydrophobic spasms. By the third day of his illness, in spite of the

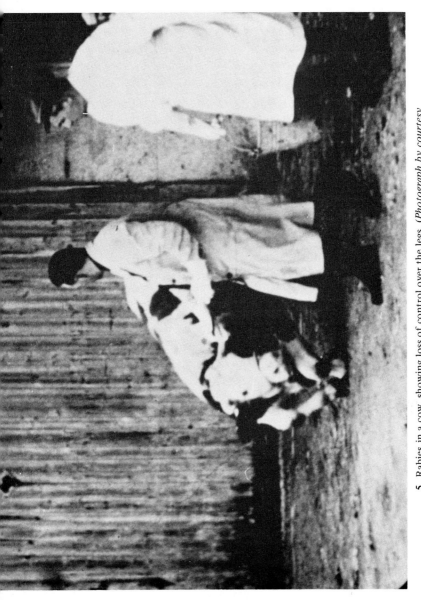

5. Rabies in a cow, showing loss of control over the legs. (*Photograph by courtesy of May and Baker Ltd*)

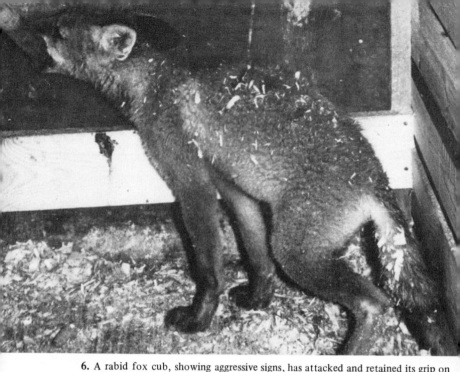

6. A rabid fox cub, showing aggressive signs, has attacked and retained its grip on a pole which was presented to it. Early signs of weakness in the hind legs are apparent.

7. Paralytic rabies in a fox, showing paralysis of legs, and staring eyes.

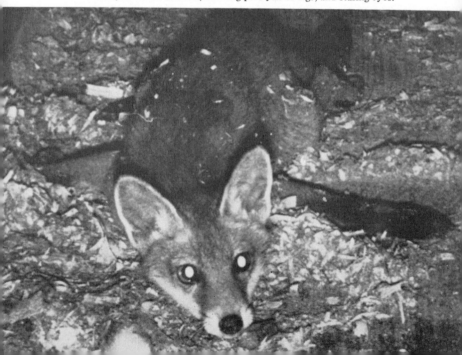

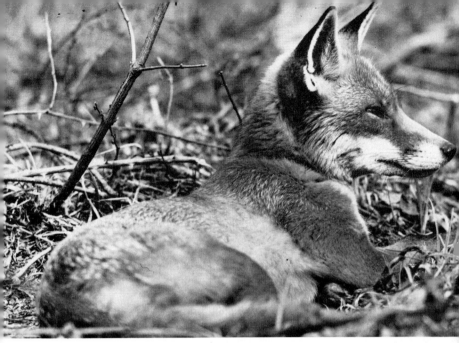

8. The red fox is widespread throughout the northern hemisphere and is both a victim and a vector of rabies throughout its range. Its generalized anatomy and behaviour together with its keen senses (look at the eyes, ears, and nose) all contribute to the fox's ability to exploit different habitats and prey. (*Photograph by D.W. Macdonald*)

9. The popular idea of the fox has been of a solitary, antisocial animal. Recent research casts doubt on this notion: the two young vixens pictured here may well grow up and spend the whole of their lives together as residents in the same territory. A correct understanding of the details of fox behaviour and ecology are crucial prerequisites for any rabies control scheme. (*Photograph by D.W. Macdonald*)

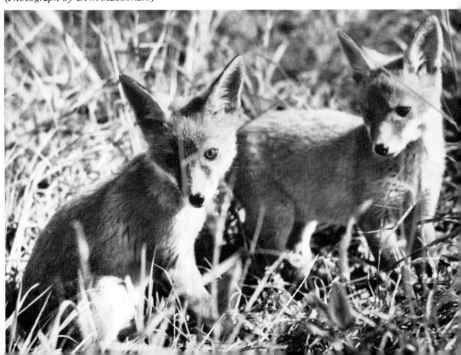

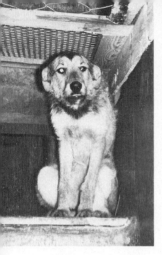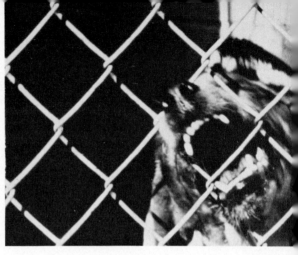

10 (above left). After a period of excitation, during which this dog barked and howled, it became depressed, shifted its weight continuously from one foreleg to the other, and sat down and rose repeatedly. The eyes became sunken and the fore teeth prominent following paralysis of the lower jaw. The dog swallowed repeatedly, making smacking noises, but there was no salivation, and it generally gave the impression of having a bone stuck in its throat. (Report from Dr. J. Müller of Copenhagen.)

11 (above right). A dog with furious rabies savagely biting the bars of its cage. (*Photograph courtesy of May and Baker Ltd*)

12. A dog showing characteristic signs of rabies. Note the dilation of the pupils, squint, drooping of the lower jaw, salivation and abnormal position of limbs.

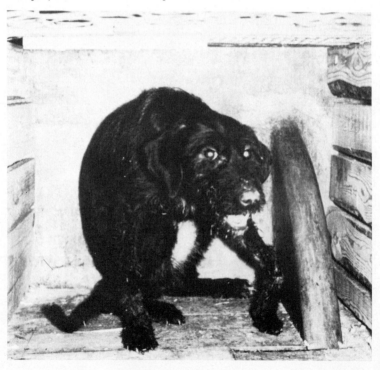

Britain. Therefore, it is of the utmost importance that cases should be recognized without delay in order to minimize the risk of transmission to other animals and, indeed, to the people in contact with the infected animal.

A common mistake is to imagine that rabies starts with, or is invariably associated with, outbursts of furious madness. Usually the first sign to be noticed in dogs is a change in temperament. Dogs that are normally friendly tend to seek solitude and creep under furniture or beds. They soon become restless, however, and move to other places of seclusion. Sudden bursts of excessive affection are commonly seen at this stage, and an afflicted animal may make persistent attempts to lick the face and hands of those persons to whom it is attached. The saliva of rabid dogs often contains virus a few days before the onset of symptoms; so this behaviour is obviously fraught with danger, especially if there are any abrasions of the skin.

There may be mild fever at the commencement of the reaction but usually this is not marked and does not persist. Gradually over a period of one to three days the symptoms become more severe. The appetite may at first be voracious but it soon wanes and may become depraved in those animals that develop the furious form of the disease. In some cases the site of the original infection suddenly becomes excessively itchy, and the dog may show an irresistible tendency to scratch and bite at the now healed wound. The pupils dilate, giving the eye a bright, glinting appearance. Salivation is increased.

The bark changes early in the course of the disease and the animal may howl in a peculiar hoarse way. When rabid dogs fight they seldom make the usual snarling noises. This change of voice was considered so characteristic of the disease that it was commonly known as a 'rabies howl'. A sudden change in the familiar voice of a dog to a throaty howl should at once act as a warning that this could be a case of rabies. The animal may show bouts of irritability, especially when disturbed, and may snap at any one, or any other animal, that comes near, or even at imaginary objects. However, even those dogs that develop the furious form of rabies usually recognize and respond to the voices of people for whom they have great affection. Such dogs seldom attack unless held tightly.

About 25 per cent of infected dogs, particularly young ones infected with the European form of rabies, may develop the furious form and show the classical symptoms associated with the popular conception of the 'mad dog'. During this stage of mental derangement, which may last a few days, the animals usually leave home and travel many miles — twenty-five or more — and attack human beings and animals including other dogs, cats, horses, cattle, sheep, etc. during their wanderings. They appear to have no feeling of pain and may bite savagely at objects such as metal bars, and will even bite themselves. The appetite often becomes depraved and they bite at and swallow, or attempt to swallow, strange objects such as stones, wood, carpets, or any other object they see. Severe constipation is often noticed. Thirst is increased and, although they may have difficulty in swallowing, at no time do these dogs or, indeed, those suffering from the paralytic form of the disease show any fear of water, the so-called 'hydrophobia' so frequently observed when human beings are affected. In spite of the severe mental derangement of dogs showing the furious form of rabies, many return, usually in a dilapidated state, to their homes. Even at this advanced stage of the disease they recognize their masters and seem to be calmed by their voices. While they seldom attack those they know, they may nevertheless snap at hands and arms if any attempt is made to restrain them, and so must be treated with great circumspection even by their owners. Usually the period of hyperexcitability is not pronounced and may be limited to such signs as excessive friendliness and perhaps sexual arousal.

Dumb rabies is characterized by the progressive development of paralysis, most marked during the early stages in the muscles of the head and neck and later in the hind limbs; periods of excitation are short or imperceptible. The eyelids tend to drop and the jaw sags. Swallowing is difficult with the result that if the animal tries to eat objects often fall from its mouth. Drinking is difficult but no signs of hydrophobia have been observed except in man. Salivation is increased in the early stages of the disease and, because of the difficulty in swallowing, the reaction may be mistaken for that produced by a bone stuck in the throat. Paralysis of the muscles is progressive but may be uneven in its distribution with the result that the dog may hold its head to one side and may turn in circles. Most sway on the hind legs. Eventually the animal goes down, becomes comatose and dies, presumably as a result of respiratory paralysis.

Many cases of rabies are not noticed until the disease is well advanced, by which time the symptoms may bear little resemblance to the classical descriptions. In the terminal stages dogs may be emaciated with sunken, often bloodshot, eyes and deceptively docile until handled.

Whether or not an infected dog develops the furious form of rabies seems to depend to some extent on the strain of virus with which it was infected. Under urban conditions the survival of the virus depends largely on infected dogs moving out of the isolation of households and actively attacking new hosts. In this way strains of virus with the propensity to produce this type of reaction are evolved by a process of natural selection.

Natural selection seems also to have produced strains of virus which are uniquely suited for survival under very specialized conditions in certain parts of the world. Thus in the arid regions of Southern Africa known as the 'sand-veld', where colonies of mongooses live in close proximity to each other in burrows, a strain of rabies virus has persisted certainly as long as records have been kept. Apart from the mongoose other free-living animals may be affected, including ground squirrels and genets as well as cattle and dogs on farms and in towns; yet the disease has remained localized over the years in these areas, partly because with the exception of Cape wild cats the disease is generally not of the furious type and the animals do not wander far.

Similary in West Africa a distinct form of rabies has existed in dogs for many years. The disease is known locally as 'oulou fato' and was identified as a form of rabies in 1912. This variant is reported to have a short incubation period − as little as seven days − and is characterized by diarrhoea and a progressive paralysis with no furious episodes. In West Africa and also in Ethiopia, it has been reported that many cases recover and that repeated attacks at long intervals may occur.

However, it should be remembered that until recently accurate diagnosis of rabies was possible only when tissue taken *post mortem* was available. Therefore, diagnosis made in the live animal must always be subject to doubt (but see Chapter 1, page 5 for recent methods of diagnosis). The blood of live animals can be examined for antibodies, but their presence may indicate no more than that the animal was in the incubation period of the disease or that it was an abortive case. An abortive case is considered to be one in which the virus does not reach the brain or if it does, does not multiply freely there. Such cases are not uncommon when small doses of virus enter the body in some place far removed from the brain, such as the leg.

The usual practice when a dog is presented for examination for rabies is to hold it in confinement for up to ten days, with the expectation that if it does have rabies it will die in about three or four days. Diagnosis can then be confirmed on tissues taken *post mortem*. While this is satisfactory in the usual type of urban rabies, it has been reported that with strains such as those found in West Africa animals may survive at least twenty-two days. Recent clinical descriptions of rabies in England are to be found in the State Veterinary Journal of 1970 in which the disease in the now famous Camberley dog 'Fritz' and another dog 'Whiskey' which had been held in quarantine in the same kennels is described.

'It was not until 10th October, 1969, six days after release from quarantine that anything untoward was noticed, when Fritz hid under a bed and howled. He also seemed stiff in his hind quarters. This was put down to unaccustomed exercise after being cooped up in quarantine kennels. On 11th October Fritz refused both food and water. Major Hemsley, who had been away for a few days, returned on 12th October and the dog came out to greet him after some encouragement, but immediately went back into hiding under the bed, being very unwilling to leave his retreat. The dog ate a little food but still refused to drink. On 13th October Fritz seemed very excitable, tending to bite in an aggressive manner in place of a friendly nibbling, and barking in a different voice. Mrs. Hemsley was in the habit of taking her own and other children to school in her car and on the morning of the 13th took the dog with her in the car. When she brought it back she put it in its basket but it persisted in barking and howling and she thought the dog was 'odd'. About 7.30. a.m. on the 14th October Major Hemsley got up as usual and let the dog out into the back garden, which was fenced in. On looking out of his bedroom window, about a quarter of an hour later, he was surprised to see Fritz in the next door garden, which was not accessible from the garden of the Hemsley's house. He also noted that Fritz was having great difficulty in defaecation and appeared terribly constipated. Major Hemsley went next door to recover his dog, when he was told by the occupant that Fritz had just killed his cat and that the milkman, who had evidently let the dog out of the Hemsley's garden, had had the sole of his boot bitten through. Fritz had disappeared. Suddenly the idea that the dog could be rabid came to Mrs. Hemsley and she realised that she must do something urgently before the dog bit anybody else. She went out at once to look for Fritz, asking her husband to seek the advice of Major Morgan Jones MRCVS who happened to live 2 doors away. Major Morgan Jones, realizing the dangers involved, advised the immediate recapture of the dog and locking it up. At 8.35 a.m. Mrs. Hemsley spotted the dog jumping into a taxi full of schoolchildren. She managed to get the dog out of the taxi, although by now it appeared to be completely mad and was furiously trying to get back into the taxi amongst the children. Mrs. Hemsley bravely hung on to the dog, calling for help. A passer-by produced a piece of string which was tied round the dog's muzzle, and Mrs. Hemsley, firmly clutching the dog to herself, walked back to the house, leaving her own car where she had stopped it. She had been bitten on the leg and arm. She took the dog to Major Morgan Jones for his advice and help. Major Morgan Jones shut it immediately in his downstairs lavatory and telephoned the Divisional Veterinary Officer to report suspected disease.'

Subsequently Major Morgan Jones stated 'It remained so in my WC for a period of some three hours. I observed the animal through the window whereupon it adopted the typical cheeky inquiring look (ears cocked, head on one side) of the typical terrier. When the kennelman came to take the dog away it showed no emotion other than a faint interest but when the dog catcher noose was applied the dog went berserk, squealing, squirming and urinating. Its facial muscles at once adopted the characteristic worried expression which did not change until the dog was taken away. My last view was of it with its face pressed close to the wire of the container cage still with the facial muscles in a state of tonus.'

Whiskey on the other hand underwent a typical dumb reaction which was recorded as follows —

Day one
Marked lethargy and depression; the eyes had a slightly vague or vacant look. There was difficulty in co-ordinating movements which were slow and unsteady. There were continuous tremors of the shoulder muscles and rhythmic movements of the left foreleg. The head was inclined to the right about 10 degrees and the lower right eyelid had dropped slightly, revealing the red conjunctiva. Periods of panting occurred. Unsuccessful attempts were made to lap water which fell from its mouth. At one stage the dog lay under its 6 inch high heavy wooden bedboard — an unnatural and uncomfortable position and one difficult for a dog of this size to attain. The dog defaecated normally at 8.30. a.m. but not again during the day. There was no evidence of micturition.

Day two
Whiskey drank about two-thirds of a bowl of water during the night and during this time it succeeded in moving its bedboard, weighing about $1\frac{1}{2}$ cwt, 2 feet across its pen. There were periods of restlessness, lying down and getting up alternating with bouts of panting. The lethargy and depression, vacant look and slow unsteady uncoordinated movements continued. The tremor was noticeable on the neck as well as the shoulders. The tilt of the head was less marked, say 5 degrees, and the right eye was half covered by the third eyelid. There was no change in the paralysis of the lower right eyelid. There was a slight paralysis or lack of tone of the muscle on the right side of the head resulting in a flattening of the parietal muscles and a dropped appearance to the right side of the face when looked at squarely. The right jowl was lower than the left. Slight salivation was occurring. The dog was able to smell, see movement and hear. It neither ate nor drank and no faeces or urine were passed.

Day three
The dog appeared a little brighter. The same general symptoms were present, but it was slightly more active and fluent in movement. Some wasting was apparent. The left lower eyelid now sagged slightly and the right eye was half closed. The conjunctivae were congested. The paralysis of the right side of the head was less apparent, possibly because both sides had become affected. The lower jaw was hanging a little open and the slight salivation continued. The dog attempted to take food and water but what little entered the mouth fell out again almost immediately. On 2 occasions the dog backed away suddenly from food and water for no apparent reason and it stood with its head facing into a corner of the pen for a short while. It could obviously see and hear.'

Cats

Cats are highly susceptible to rabies but because they tend to live a solitary existence they are unlikely to serve as reservoirs of infection.

Nevertheless, rabid cats present a serious problem since about 75 per cent of those that succumb to the disease become highly aggressive. Because of this tendency and because they are relatively easy to hide they could well be responsible for the introduction of the disease into controlled areas.

Young male cats which by nature are adventurous and aggressive are more frequently affected than others. The early stages of the disease in cats are not readily discernible but, as in other animals, the disease starts with change in behaviour, including loss of appetite, restlessness, and excessive friendliness. These changes are accompanied by difficulty in swallowing and so the cat may drool as paralysis increases. In most cases periods of aggression soon develop and the animal may scratch or bite without provocation. The furious form of rabies shown by most rabid cats can be very frightening to watch. During paroxysms the eyes flash, the mouth foams, the back arches, and the claws are protruded. Determined efforts are made to attack any person or animal that approaches and, as a cat launches its attacks at its victim's head, they are particularly dangerous. As in the case of other animals the cry is usually altered. Unlike dogs, however, rabid cats seldom recognize their owners and do not respond to their voices. The period of excitement usually lasts two to four days but may be as short as twenty-four hours. Gradually signs of progressive paralysis become more apparent and the animals usually die in three or four days, but occasionally up to 8 days after the onset of symptoms.

The few cats (about 25 per cent) that show the dumb form of the disease usually die in a day or two after showing no more than progressive paralysis accompanied by spells of excessive affection and constant purring.

Horses

When horse-drawn vehicles and rabid dogs roamed the streets of Europe towards the end of the last century, cases of rabies in horses were not uncommon. Now that the horse has virtually disappeared from the streets and rabies in dogs is largely under control cases are rare; a history of exposure is not usually available, but when it is, the fox has always been incriminated as the vector. The great majority of cases probably resulted from fox bites while the animals were out at pasture, but the possibility that some could be infected when stabled should not be forgotten, since it is known that rabid foxes lose their fear of man and show a tendency to enter buildings.

Like cattle, horses are highly inquisitive animals and frequently nuzzle any animal showing unusual behaviour. They are thus prone to bites on the lips and muzzle, with the result that few fail to react. The incubation period is seldom longer than six weeks. In Europe the disease usually runs a rapid course. The animals may die within 24 hours, and few survive more than four days.

The symptoms vary from animal to animal. The minority develop the paralytic form of the disease, but most have an agonising death. As in other animals the first signs are changes in behaviour accompanied by a mild rise in temperature. The victim becomes anxious, and mental aberration gradually increases to a state of marked agitation. Sexual excitment may be intense. The upper lips are drawn back baring the teeth, and wrinkling the nose and lips. Rabid horses appear to be thirsty but cannot swallow. They shake their heads violently, foam at the mouth, grind their teeth and whinney frequently as if in great pain, lie down, stand up, sit like a dog, strain in futile attempts to pass dung, may lash out wildly with their hind legs, and show signs of severe colic. Although they will usually bite at anything such as a stick thrust at them, they do not show aggression, but may show a marked antipathy to dogs. Finally they go down and are unable to rise. At this time they may thrash about with their feet. Muscle spasms are rarely seen.

Unless the animal was seen to have been bitten diagnosis is uncertain on clinical signs, but rabies should be suspected if exposure was possible.

There is regulated but fairly free passage of horses between Europe and the United Kingdom. A period in quarantine is not required. Theoretically rabies could be introduced in this way but because the horses concerned are kept under close supervision the chance is considered remote. The chance of a rabid horse spreading the disease to animals other than man is negligible.

Cattle

In those countries where the disease is endemic in wildlife, rabies is of frequent occurrence in cattle. Thus in France the number of cases reported in cattle is second only to those in the fox. Among 2881 cases recorded there from March 1968 to May 1973 there were 2722 in foxes, 697 in cattle, 127 in cats, 105 in dogs, 59 in badgers and 34 in roe deer. Cattle which remain outdoors especially at night are most vulnerable to attack. Because of their innate curiosity and because they tend to defend their territory against marauders, cattle are prone to bites on the muzzle by rabid animals. As they are highly susceptible to rabies few fail to react and in Europe the incubation period is seldom prolonged. Cattle infected by vampire bats in South America react in a similar manner but the incubation period may be much longer.

At first no more than vague signs of mental disturbance are seen. The cattle are somewhat depressed and usually the milk yield is reduced. Gradually the symptoms become more obvious. Muscular tremors are often seen and there is increased salivation. Because paralysis of the swallowing muscles is usually pronounced, the animals tend to slobber and gulp and have difficulty in drinking water. As in the dog, however, there is no hydrophobia or fear of water. So marked are these signs in some animals that the condition is commonly diagnosed as obstruction of the gullet. Anyone attempting to search manually for any obstacle in such cases is, of course, liable to infection through abrasions caused by contact with the animal's teeth.

In some cases cattle become highly excited, bellow incessantly in an altered voice and, bulls especially, may show marked sexual excitement. Their eyes become wild and staring. Many animals groan continuously with apparent colic. Some may develop a tendency to attack other animals and man. These attacks, which may also be made on inanimate objects such as trees, are usually made with the horns and may be so fierce that it is not unusual for a horn to be broken. Because cattle seldom bite, transmission to other animals is rare.

The animals usually stop eating fairly early in the course of the disease but some may show depraved appetite and attempt to eat unusual objects such as stones or bits of wood. Constipation followed by diarrhoea may be seen. Knuckling over at the fetlocks may be one of the first symptoms. The disease usually lasts four to seven days during which the animals lose weight and show signs of progressive paralysis of all muscles, but especially of the hind legs which induces a swaying gait. Eventually they collapse and usually become comatose shortly before death.

The signs shown by cattle are clearly illustrated in a graphic description made in 1844, at a time when considerable attention was paid to the symptomatology of disease, since accurate diagnosis depended entirely on the astuteness of the observer and not on laboratory tests as it does now. Here follows an extract from the report made at the time.

'The affected animals ran with tossed-up heads and wild looks madly round the pastures, goring and striking at all other animals with their horns. Every now and again the upper lip was drawn upwards in that peculiar manner in which vicious animals are apt to twitch it, and they kept up a continuous bellowing, which struck all hearers with terror, and which was not excited by the sight of a dog or any other creature, though it increased it. They foamed at the mouth; the hind parts were weak and the weakness increased so rapidly that on the third day the animals were usually stretched on the ground, and could not be raised but with great difficulty. The muscles of the thighs, shoulders, and face were contracted at intervals as by spasms; and if the cattle chanced to be tied up they were restless, gazed wildly about, and bellowed frequently; if free, they rushed straight onwards over everything until some obstacle impeded their progress and then they fell heels-over-head and lay still, apparently exhausted. There was no unusual thirst, and the power to swallow remained unimpaired. Any fluids poured in the mouth, as water, bran gruel etc., were sucked down, and the only peculiarity observable was a motion as of choking, and a twitching of the muscles of the face. The disease was very fatal, most of the affected animals dying about the end of the fourth day.'

Pigs

In an outbreak of rabies that was observed in a herd of pigs all the affected animals showed twitching of the snout, rapid chewing movements, and excessive salivation followed by convulsions. They died a day or two after the onset of the disease. A remarkable feature of the disease in these pigs was that they could not be made to squeal.

Sheep

In sheep, rabies usually starts with depression of movements and appetite. Soon, however, periods of agitation may ensue during which sexual excitement may be a spectacular feature of the disease; this is considered by some to be the most commonly seen symptom. During paroxysms the eyes are staring with dilated pupils, the nose runs, and the animals may slobber at the mouth. Rams especially grind their teeth and butt anything they see, including other sheep, dogs, human beings, or trees, and it is not unusual for them to attempt to bite, but because they lack upper incisor and canine teeth they seldom cause wounds. Rabid sheep are usually silent, but may occasionally bleat in a strange low-pitched bellow.

After the period of excitement, which may sometimes be absent, the animals become dull, lie down, and show a copious flow of saliva and nasal secretions. Death usually follows five to eight days after the start of symptoms.

Recent reports of rabies in sheep are rare, but there is one by Dr Darbyshire who observed an outbreak in Rhodesia in 1953 while he was stationed there. This outbreak had the characteristics of the disease as seen in Europe.

'The owner informed the Department of Veterinary Services locally that he suspected rabies in a number of his sheep. The farm was visited soon afterwards the same day and a flock of some 150 Merino sheep were seen together in a pen. The owner contended that a number of them had been bitten by a honey badger 20 days previously, and he reported that the native herd-boy had noticed that a number of them seemed to be excited the previous evening. The sheep had accordingly been penned up overnight.

'Eventually 11 sheep were chosen from the flock as showing abnormal behaviour. In addition, one sheep had been found dead not far from the homestead. Two others were lying in a comatose condition outside the pen. In one of the latter there was profuse salivation. The respiratory rate was rapid and shallow in both. The eyes were closed and both showed opisthotonus [arched back].

'Of the 11 chosen from the flock, one ewe was reported to have been chewing the wool of one of the lambs, and on examination appeared very excited. Between intervals of comparative rest, during which it displayed twitching at the lips, general restlessness, and excitability, it was aggressive towards its companions. This was the only real case of aggressiveness among the affected animals. There was no excessive salivation in this animal. Another ewe salivated profusely and suffered from dyspnoea [laboured breathing]. When handled, it fell to the ground as if exhausted and lay for several minutes on its side before attempting to rise. The remainder of the animals chosen exhibited a general restlessness, abnormal sexual behaviour and excitement, demonstrated by riding each other continuously, twitching the lips, and wild staring eyes. In all, 40 animals appeared to have definite but healed wounds, as if from being bitten, on the face and forelegs, including all those 11 sheep picked out. No bleating was heard [contrast the frequent bellowing often observed in rabid cattle], and there was no apparent irritation or itching of the scars of these wounds.

'In all, 47 sheep died, with three cases diagnosed as positive in the laboratory and 44 clinical cases. Of these, 14 commenced to show clinical symptoms after being bitten on the face by a badger 19 days previously. A further 19 showed obvious clinical symptoms 25 days after being bitten and were destroyed, and seven had died after showing symptoms for a period of five to six days. One animal died a week after commencing to show symptoms. It is of interest to note that when the 19 were destroyed, seven others were not showing sufficient symptoms to warrant destruction, but nevertheless they died the next day. A further seven sheep showed clinical symptoms 27 days after being bitten.'

Deer

Deer are as prone to rabies as cattle and show similar symptoms. Therefore it is not surprising that during the recent epizooty in Europe a number of cases have been reported, particularly in roe deer.

Before the eradication of rabies in Britain at the turn of the century, deer confined to parks were highly vulnerable to attack by wandering dogs suffering from the furious form of rabies. Most noteworthy was the outbreak in Richmond Park reported in 1887 by the Department of Agriculture when out of a total of about 1200 animals in the park 257, mostly fallow deer, died of rabies. As it is the custom of these animals to congregate in small herds which rarely mingle, it is apparent that the incidence in individual groups must have been very high.

Experiments made then proved that the disease could be transmitted from one deer to another by animals that showed signs of the furious form of the disease. However, it was apparent that, in the field, transmission of this sort occurred too rarely to maintain the infection in a herd, in the absence of rabid dogs.

There is probably no better description of the disease in deer than that contained in the Ministry Report issued at the time.

The earliest symptom observed in most cases was that of throwing their heads back on the shoulders and keeping their noses pointed to the sky; the animals were then seen to make sudden starts and gallop right away from the rest of the herd.

Next they began to rush at other deer, also at posts, rails, trees, or other fixed objects. When rushing at the latter they bruised their heads between the horns and rubbed off the hair in patches. This may be looked upon as a prominent sign in the early stages of the disease. [Note that this sign must not be confused with the 'normal' loss of hair between the antlers of sika deer.]

Subsequently, instead of being timid, they became unusually bold, charging at other deer, and causing the greatest alarm in the herd, and if kept in close confinement they would rush at persons or objects brought in their way. At times a fawn might be seen to pursue and bite at old deer in a manner quite unnatural.

After a few days' illness the animals invariably died, some presenting violent paroxysms, while in other instances paralysis of the limbs became most marked before death.

Foxes

Now that rabies in dogs can be controlled by the strict application of sanitary measures, including elimination of stray dogs and cats, accompanied by muzzling and vaccination of registered dogs, wild animals are left as the main reservoirs of infection, especially in Europe and North America (see Chapter 1 for a discussion of the epizootiology of the disease in these continental areas.)

Foxes are classed among the animals most highly susceptible to rabies and are especially so when the virus to which they are exposed has been selected by passage from fox to fox. When infected in laboratory trials with fox strains of virus, few survive more than three to four days after the onset of symptoms, though occasionally cubs may last ten days. Not all foxes that have been exposed to rabies develop symptoms of the disease. In infected areas a number of apparently normal foxes are found which have antibodies to the disease indicating that the virus has entered their bodies; some of these could be incubating the disease but others presumably received small doses of virus in parts of the body such as the feet or tail and this has failed to reach the brain.

The symptoms shown by foxes have been described in detail by American and Swiss workers both from laboratory trials and from observations made by farmers in the country-side. As in other animals the disease in foxes may be divided into three phases i.e. change in temperament, excitation, and finally paralysis. Early in the course of the disease the animals become restless, the voice changes to what has been termed a 'yowl' very different from the characteristic howl or bark of foxes. The pupils become dilated, giving the eye a glinting appearance. Rabid foxes lose all sense of direction and as this is accompanied by a loss of fear of man or animals they frequently wander some miles into out-buildings, garages, or even homesteads. (It is worth remembering, however, that occasionally even normal foxes will enter buildings.)

The furious form is seldom seen, but foxes may be aggressive and make unprovoked attacks on men or animals, or they may bite inanimate objects. Usually at this stage of the disease, signs of paralysis of the legs and jaws develop and the animals tend to stagger. The onset of paralysis appears to be related to the site of infection and, as in other animals, these parts may show signs of itchiness. When present the irritation is apparently not severe, for foxes seldom mutilate themselves in the way animals such as monkeys do. Even in the advanced stages of the disease foxes remain aggressive and may snap at anyone who disturbs them. Therefore it is most important that any fox which appears moribund and harmless should be treated with great caution and either killed or held in safe confinement while help is sought.

Monkeys

A case of rabies was observed in a rhesus monkey imported from India. The animal became ill 47 days after arrival in England. At no time did it show aggressive tendencies; rather it cowered in a corner of its cage continually biting its fingers and hands. So severe were these self-inflicted wounds that the animal had to be destroyed. No sign of pain was evident while the animal was biting itself. The assumption must be that it was through wounds in the monkey's hands that the virus had gained entry to the animal's body and that damage to the nerves in this area caused intensive itching and irritation.

Other animals

Besides the animals specifically mentioned above, rabies in Europe has been reported in poultry — rare, though, since few birds survive the initial attack — and in a number of wild animals including badgers, martens, polecats, weasels, bats and rodents. Of these only the polecat in Europe seems to be a potential reservoir of infection and even then only in very localized areas. However, it should be recognized that all those animals with well-formed incisors capable of inflicting wounds are potentially dangerous, and in no circumstances should a wild animal which appears tame and friendly be handled.

The role of bats as vectors of rabies has been well documented in America. However, cases in European bats are rare, and the bat does not at this stage appear to be of importance as a vector. The possibility of an infected bat flying across the Channel is more than remote.

The claim that wild rodents in Eastern Europe harbour, without showing signs of disease, a 'rabies-like' virus which on passage through susceptible animals produces a disease indistinguishable from rabies, should be accepted with caution. This is discussed more fully in Chapter 1.

Recently, mink which have escaped from fur-producing ranches in various parts of Britain have been shown to be capable of breeding in the free state. There is the potential danger here that rabies might enter this country and become enzootic in mink much in the way it has become established in the mongoose which was introduced into the West Indian Islands to control snakes and rodents. The mongoose is now a greater scourge on the islands than the snakes ever were. Far from reducing the snake population they serve as an additional source of food for the snakes and as they are now enzootically infected with rabies virus they show how dangerous it can be to introduce into a territory exotic species of animal or plant life.

Distrust then any animal which shows sudden change in temperament or voice, especially one known to have been imported into the country, even though it has served its time in quarantine. Always consider the possibility of rabies in any imported animal which develops behavioural changes.

5

The behavioural ecology
of the red fox

DAVID W. MACDONALD

Although the red fox is, by tradition, a familiar animal to the British public, its sudden proliferation through the pages of our newspapers has left many people puzzled. The popular press has pointed to a 'bushy tailed outlaw' and a new 'Red Peril' from the East, while readers of Hansard will have noted that questions concerning foxes recently reached a peak of almost thirty per month. Everyone appreciates that we face the threat of rabies and that much of continental Europe is already within the compass of the disease, but the frequently posed question is 'What's so special about foxes?'. In the course of this chapter I shall try to provide some answers to this question in the light of our present knowledge of fox biology. At the same time I shall discuss measures that have been, or may be, employed to check the spread of fox rabies in the context of our understanding of the animals' behaviour and shall attempt to convince the reader that the study of such apparent trivia as whether a particular fox spends its time eating beetles as opposed to rabbits, which may at first sight seem a purely academic occupation, is potentially crucial to the success of control schemes designed to halt the disease.

First, it is necessary to outline the form and extent of the problem. With the exception of a few isolated land masses (including the British Isles and Australia) rabies is found throughout much of the world. It seems that this has been so for a considerable time, for there are accounts of the disease from ancient civilizations of the Nile and Euphrates more than 2000 years ago. Although rabies was first described in the New World by English colonists in the eighteenth century, it may have been present for much longer, perhaps even reaching North America via the Bering land bridge over 30 000 years ago since similar symptoms have been described for generations by Eskimos. Throughout its history rabies has caused terror to human populations wherever it has occurred and many fabulous remedies have been prescribed; amongst these is a particularly longstanding preventive measure advocated by Pliny who recommended excising the so-called 'worm' under the tongue (actually the harmless tissue known as the lyssa). This

70

operation was still being performed in England at the end of the nineteenth century.

Earlier reports of the disease normally involve dogs, which remain the primary risk to man in underdeveloped countries today. Nevertheless, while overshadowed in importance to man by the risk from dogs, wildlife must have suffered from endemic (or more correctly enzootic) rabies also, for there are accounts of rabid wolves in Asia in the thirteenth century and of foxes in the United States and Europe in the eighteenth and nineteenth centuries.

In France between 1851 and 1877 there were 770 human deaths from rabies of which 707 resulted from bites from rabid dogs, 38 from wolves, 23 from cats, and 1 each from a fox and a cow. Similar figures were collected in France, Germany, Württemberg, and Italy in the late nineteenth century. Overall, during that period of history in Europe, roughly 90 per cent of people dying of rabies were infected by dogs, 4 per cent by cats, 4 per cent by wolves and 2 per cent by foxes. The changing status of rabies as a disease of humans is reflected in a comparison between those figures and present-day France where there has been only one death from rabies since 1946. Figures have been kept on the number of animals *reported* with rabies in France between March 1968 and December 1975 of which foxes represented 78·5 per cent of the total 9465 cases, with cattle coming second with 10·2 per cent. Similarly, of the 50 617 animal cases reported in the Federal Republic of Germany during the 18 years between 1954 and 1972, 63·5 per cent were foxes. Clearly foxes are a frequent *victim* of the disease.

It is interesting to compare these figures with those indicating the apparent risk to people from the various possible vectors of the disease. In West Berlin 221 people were given anti-rabies prophylactic treatment in 1965 having been bitten by potentially rabid animals, of which 149 (67·4 per cent) were dogs, 32 (14·5 per cent) were cats, 8 (3·6 per cent) were foxes, 26 (11·8 per cent) were rodents, 2 were deer, 2 were hedgehogs, and there was 1 boar and 1 marten. During the 21-year period between 1945 and 1966, 5 people died from rabies in West Germany and 32 in East Germany.

In general it seems that, irrespective of the high incidence of infected foxes, the decrease in human rabies outbreaks parallels the reduction of the disease in dogs. In Europe, with a general awareness of the risks from stray dogs, the availability of excellent post-exposure prophylaxis and the compulsory use of vaccines for pets, the dog problem has been controlled. The situation is less happy where cats are concerned. While the number of rabid dogs in the United States fell from 5688 in 1953 to 235 in 1971 (a decline of 96 per cent), the number of infected cats decreased from 538 to 222 (only 59 per cent). Similarly, of the 79 rabid domestic animals reported in Switzerland between 1967 and 1970,

40 were cats and 6 were dogs, and it was cats that caused 3 out of 23 deaths from rabies amongst people in East Germany between 1953 and 1961, and 15 out of 25 deaths in Hungary, while being the origin of 53·3 per cent of the bites treated in Potsdam between 1959 and 1964. The difficulty of controlling the independent wandering of cats remains a serious problem in the campaign against rabies in Europe and certain Swiss cantons now dictate by law that cats must be walked on leads. The trend in the United States (while being greatly complicated by the presence of other vectors amongst the wildlife such as skunks, raccoons, and bats) parallels that in Europe with a dramatic decline in canine rabies due to vaccination campaigns and a concomitant decrease in human rabies with 56 cases between 1950 and 1970 (21 caused by dogs or cats, 10 by skunks, 7 by bats, and 6 by foxes). None of the 6 deaths in America between 1970 and 1973 resulted from foxes. Even today in the United States every rabid dog or cat results in 2·4 persons receiving post-exposure treatment, while only 0·4 people require such treatment for each case of wildlife rabies reported, because of the greater risk of contact with rabid domestic animals.

It seems, then, that in Europe and North America rabies does not present a significant threat to human life. Many cases that are subjected to post-exposure treatment still result from contact with domestic animals and not foxes or other wild species. Of course, these domestic animals may, in turn, have contracted the disease from wildlife. Nevertheless, it is important to put our discussion of the fox in perspective: the threat in the United States and Europe may not be to life itself, but it certainly is to the 'quality' of life, endangering our current relaxed attitude to domestic animals and, perhaps most tragic, threatening to prejudice our relationship with wildlife and the countryside. This threat to our peace of mind in the countryside cannot be overestimated. Even in the underdeveloped world where rabies is still a human killer, it is relatively insignificant compared to, for instance, tuberculosis or malaria, but it poses an enormous threat to livestock (see Chapter 1). Rabies, as a threat to either life, economics, or 'quality' of life, is a serious problem and one which, at least for the non-tropical world, involves the fox in large numbers. Thus we must understand more about the biology of the species.

The red fox of the British Isles has an enormous geographical range within which it lives in a huge variety of contrasting habitats. The same species of fox that forages amongst the suburbs of London and in the Highlands of Scotland (themselves dramatically different environments) can also be found throughout Europe, north through Scandinavia to the Arctic Circle, eastwards to Korea, southwards to the deserts of North Africa and Arabia. The same species also spans North America, reaching up into the Canadian Arctic and down through the deserts and arid zones of New Mexico, and further into Central America. Within its geographical range the red fox overlaps with various of the twenty or so other species of fox; the Arctic fox of the north, the Fennec and Rupels foxes of Arabia, the grey fox, kit fox, and others, of the New World. The picture is clearly one of an unusually adaptable and, in that sense, successful animal. One of the first questions the designers of rabies control schemes might ask is whether the fox presents the same 'problem' in all parts of its geographical range. The answer to this, an insight into the reasons for its success as a species, can be gained from knowledge of the fox's eating habits.

Fox diet has been studied exhaustively by generations of scientists (over one hundred studies during the past fifty years), partly because it is one of the few things that can easily be studied about this elusive nocturnal creature. The analyses are based on detailed examination of either faeces or stomach contents (the latter taken from dead animals) or both. The results share one common feature: whatever the principal food may be in any given area, all foxes invariably eat a variety of very different types of food, including various small rodents, birds, rabbits, insects, fruits, and carrion. Foods range in size from beetles to the occasional hare or roe-deer fawn and it seems that whatever is available will be eaten to at least some extent. As the availability of different prey changes in any one place from season to season, so will the fox's diet change also. That is not to say that the foxes are indiscriminate feeders or hunters. On the contrary, I have recently conducted field experiments that demonstrate marked preferences for certain foods over others (for instance, relishing the field vole more than the bank vole). Nevertheless, when necessary, the fox can and does survive on a tremendous variety of foods.

The diet of the majority of the fox population of Britain has changed dramatically in the recent past with the introduction of rabbit myxomatosis. This disease was introduced into the United Kingdom in 1952 as a means of controlling a rabbit population of plague proportions. Previously two British zoologists, Southern and Watson, had conducted a study of the diet of foxes and demonstrated a heavy dependence on the rabbit. In 1959 Lever was able to follow up their work after the rabbits' numbers had crashed and found that the diet had, perforce, changed, containing many more small mammals than before. A similar change in menu was observed by the Swedish biologist, Englund, when myxomatosis was introduced to the island of Gotland for rabbit control purposes. There is evidence to show that this change in diet temporarily influenced fox numbers as well; figures from the Forestry Commission and fox clubs of Scotland have been analysed by Nature Conservancy biologists and show an increase in the number of foxes killed during 1959 (the year after myxomatosis in Scotland), presumably because of a very successful fox year consequent upon the abundance of dying and easily caught rabbits. This was, in turn, followed by a temporary decline in fox numbers in the face of a food shortage.

My own study of foxes is an attempt to relate the behaviour of the fox in any one area with the habitat conditions in that area. To that end I have carefully selected different study areas that I thought would exemplify the extremes of the fox's range and probe the limits of its flexibility. In each area I have collected faeces for analysis in the laboratory. Of more than three thousand samples of faeces examined from different areas, some, from agricultural land, conform to the general picture containing a variety of food remains from rodents, birds, fruit, and insects, while others, collected from an adjacent but different habitat, contained the remains of huge numbers of earthworms together with plenty of fruit and occasional scraps pilfered from bird-tables. While working in these two areas I was also commuting to the Fells of Cumbria where the primary food was rabbit, supplemented by voles and sheep carrion.

Each new study area discloses new prey supplies. Recently, in the Italian Alps, I have found evidence of foxes scavenging from dead chamois, while in the desert of Israel, a local population of at least ten foxes acquired more than 87 per cent of their total food intake from one piece of ground less than ten metres square where the Nature Reserves Authority maintained a feeding site regularly provisioned with offal. Around the same feeding site I watched foxes following striped hyaenas in order to pilfer from them, and in the Abbruzzo Mountains of Italy I have followed fox tracks that in turn followed wolf tracks to seek out and loot hidden caches of food left by the wolf for future use. Clearly the fox can thrive on a variety of foods that are acquired by diverse hunting techniques. A fox might be seen to break off from delicate pacing after earthworms to burst into a sprint in pursuit of a rabbit. This versatility in tastes and hunting techniques goes a long way to explaining the widespread occurrence of the fox which combines with its susceptibility to rabies to make it a victim of the disease over most of the northern hemisphere.

There is now an accumulating body of evidence that supports the intuitively obvious contention that the availability and dispersion of food will be amongst the factors determining the home range covered by an animal (home range being that area within which the daily, or nightly, routine activities of the animal occur). As foxes can contract, and in turn transmit, rabies, it is of fundamental importance to know how far and how quickly they can move and hence spread the disease. On the basis of the dramatically different diet of foxes in different areas, one might predict corresponding differences in home range size also. Any such differences could be very relevant both to the speed at which rabies spreads through a fox population and also to the considerations involved in drawing up any plans to contain the disease. Until quite recently it has been difficult to gather this type of information on foxes, again because of their elusive and nocturnal nature, and estimates of range size (and total population density) have been based on inspired guesswork or hearsay. In the face of these practical difficulties, researchers have concentrated on 'populations' rather than 'individuals'.

Several studies have been conducted in which cubs (and adults) are captured around breeding earths, fitted with numbered ear-tags and then released. Later the ear-tags are recovered from hunters (sometimes under the incentive of a bounty) and a measure is taken of the straight-line distance between the original point of capture and the point of recovery. Nothing is known about what happened between these two points nor about the route taken. Some of these studies have involved huge numbers of foxes and yielded valuable information on their dispersal. Amongst the records are some phenomenal long-distance treks, one of 257 km (160 miles) and one of 394 km (245 miles), but these are very exceptional and the majority travel only short distances: three American studies showed that for males, as opposed to females, the average distances travelled before being killed were 43, 26, and 26·3 km, and for females 8, 13·3, and 7·1 km. The differences between these results assuredly relate to differences in the behaviour and ecology of the fox populations under study, the details of which cannot be resolved using this type of technique alone.

In Britain Gwyn Lloyd has conducted a similar study on 272 marked cubs in two different habitats in Wales. In one of these, a sheep farming area in the hills, males travelled an average of 10·4 km to females 2·2. In another area, where the population density was presumed to be much higher, the respective distances were males 4·6 and females 1·9 km. These areas also differ in the mean age of tagged cubs on recovery (8·5 months:18·6 months). This illustrated a difficulty for all such studies in that it is impossible to standardize the hunting practices, perseverance, and honesty of the hunters, all of which can appreciably affect results. By their nature these studies concern large areas of land which may cover various different habitat types, regions of hunting intensity, and so forth. The 'average fox' which emerges from such information may correspond only remotely with a real individual. Nevertheless, perhaps the important point to be remembered is that the differences do exist between results from different areas and between the sexes, and that these need to be explored. Such differences may result from aspects of the fox's biology that affect its role in rabies outbreaks and should affect our counterplans.

Recent studies have tried to overcome shortcomings of the ear-tagging technique by complementing this coarse grain data with detailed information on the movements of given individuals by radio tracking. This has been done in America, in several European countries, and in Britain by Gwyn Lloyd and myself. My own work has been an effort to provide fine grain information on relatively few individuals which could be married up with diet and habitat analyses done in the same areas. To this end I have radio-tagged and followed the movements of over sixty foxes in diverse habitats. My radio collars (miniature transmitters fitted on a collar to the fox's neck, each of which emits bleeps on a different channel) give out a signal which can be received up to six miles away. Following the animals at night I do not use this equipment as an end in itself as it can only yield information on the approximate position of the fox whilst my interest is knowing not only where the fox is, but also what it is doing there and why. I use the radio to attempt to stalk the fox until I am in a position to watch it with a pair of infra-red binoculars which permit moderately good vision in complete darkness while I remain undetected by the animal. Even with these sophisticated pieces of equipment the problems of following the fox are many; a change in wind direction or a snapped twig can still ruin hours of careful stalking. Nevertheless, the major hurdle of being unable to see at night has been substantially lowered and when the animal is in sight there can be no question about the accuracy of the observation.

Information is starting to accumulate from radio tracking and one review of various studies in America quotes the wide spectrum of home range sizes from 259 to 777 hectares (1 hectare = 100 metres X 100 metres = 10 000 square metres), which means that some ranges can be three times the area of others. However, by attempting to work in areas at the different extremes of food availability, I have found range sizes beyond these limits, varying between less than 30 hectares and more than 1300 hectares. That is to say that there are stable fox home ranges in different parts of England that vary in size by a factor of well over forty. To make these measurements a bit easier to visualize it might be helpful to remember that the grounds of a football stadium measure about one hectare.

These figures for home range size apply to both dog foxes and vixens and raise the question of how this is compatible with the differences in straightline movements mentioned above that exist between sexes in the ear-tagging studies. This paradox is a consequence of social divisions within the fox population which, as with many other animal populations, falls into at least two sections: resident and non-resident individuals. The former have a fixed home range from which they seldom, if ever, venture and it is to this stable category that the above radio tracking figures apply. The non-resident category is composed of animals who have apparently been unable to establish themselves in home ranges and disperse over unpredictable routes on unknown ground. Figures provided by the ear-tagging recoveries lump together permanent residents and dispersing foxes of both sexes, in addition to some that may have changed status from one category to another during the intervening time.

To understand the role played by foxes in the spread of rabies it is necessary to disentangle the mechanisms underlying the behaviour of both resident and itinerant sections of the population. While the home range size and frontiers of foxes resident within my study areas have remained remarkably constant throughout my investigation, this is almost certainly not true in areas suffering repeated and serious disturbance in the form of human depredations on foxes. It seems that dispersing foxes can be found at most times of the year, but they are most in evidence during the winter months from September to February, when not only the many young of the preceding spring leave their parents' range, but also a number of older males cover relatively large distances, presumably in search of home ranges of their own. Both male and female cubs may disperse from their parents' range, but in different numbers and to different extents. For instance, one American study showed that of animals tagged as cubs but killed before they were two years old, 96 per cent of the males had moved more than eight km while only 58 per cent of the vixens had moved this distance. Again, other studies obtained different results, but the general finding is that a smaller proportion of female cubs leave their natal area than of males. Those vixens that do leave, do not travel so far as their brothers. During the same months of the year that this movement takes place the resident animals remain within their customary ranges.

Radio tracking of dispersing foxes by Storm, an American zoologist, has revealed that five young dogs averaged fifteen km per night over a fourteen-night period during which three young vixens averaged nine km per night. Both sexes moved in roughly straight lines (contrasting markedly with the interwoven movements of resident foxes) but veered occasionally to avoid major obstructions such as lakes and rivers. Amongst the tracks of male foxes of varying ages that I have followed at this season there have also been long straight movements at fair speed, but these are often interspersed with periods of several days in one small area and the long runs of successive nights may criss-cross back and forwards across the same general locality. This, together with the fact that several radio-tagged dog foxes have on occasion congregated in one residential range, leads me to suspect that at least part of the pattern results from homing-in on receptive vixens.

Of course, the extent to which individual animals are in contact and to which they are travelling across different pieces of land, hugely influences the possibilities of disease transmission. Indeed, rabies shows a seasonal peak in outbreaks of the disease amongst foxes which coincides with the winter period of cub dispersal and the long-range movements of males. We do not know the extent to which these changing movement patterns influence the frequency of social inter-action in normal foxes (far less rabid ones). In the absence of firm observational reports, attempts have been made using a computer to simulate the movement patterns typical of resident and dispersing foxes to gauge the probability of encounters between them in different circumstances (for instance with different population densities). As yet such attempts cannot be backed up with sufficient field data to be really instructive; we do not know, for instance, the extent to which a resident seeks contact with an intruder, nor vice versa, nor is it clear from what distance they can sense each other's presence, nor how this differs between healthy and rabid animals. The picture with healthy animals is, however, becoming clearer; on several occasions I have watched, with infra-red binoculars, as a dispersing male crossed the range of a radio-tagged resident and the resident chased him vigorously, and if this is general then the rate of contact would be extremely high. Another problem that remains, rather like that of where flies go in the winter, is where these surplus animals go in summer. Huge numbers are killed annually and I have some scanty evidence suggesting that others keep moving over a relatively enormous, but more regular area. The details await more research and could considerably influence our opinion of the seasonal risk of rabies transmission.

There is yet a third category of movements: these are the occasional excursions made by established residents out of their range. These trips, while not frequently undertaken, seem common to all foxes (although perhaps more so amongst males than females) and normally involve a swift excursion straight to and back from some particularly bountiful food source. Those excursions that I have witnessed have commonly taken place very late at night, suggesting to me that they were motivated by an unsuccessful night's foraging. This idea has been supported by field experiments, when tame, but free ranging radio-collared foxes have also made similar trips from their normal haunts when I failed to feed them as usual. If this explanation is correct, then such trips might be more frequent in areas where the fox's diet was not only unpredictable, but where there were localized supplies of super-abundant food that could be tapped in an emergency. A Dutch student of fox biology, Niewold, has described excursions to a particularly rewarding caravan site and also to the rich feeding sites provided for wild boar by hunters. As these trips constitute a departure from the normal confined movements of resident foxes, they might increase the possibility of disease transmission during the otherwise less hazardous summer months.

The behavioural ecology of the red fox

Already it can be seen that the fox (and hence its control or manipulation) presents a very different proposition from one area to the next (even neighbouring areas) and that the simple question that an innocent health official might ask, such as 'How far do foxes travel?' cannot evoke a simple unqualified answer, but probes both a profoundly complicated issue, and fields of study which are in their infancy for all animals, especially the elusive fox. Furthermore, there is another factor to consider, namely, how are these home ranges (of whatever dimensions they may be) arranged in space? Do they overlap each other or are they defended against neighbouring foxes and hence do they constitute territories (defined as a defended area)? To answer this we begin to explore the social organization of the fox.

The most striking feature of accumulated radio tracking data gathered within my principal study area, is that the land is divided into a number of non-overlapping fox ranges. By watching with the infra-red binoculars I have witnessed a number of fights between neighbouring residents that suggest that these ranges are vigorously defended along their borders. Of course, such fights are rare because there are other and less energetic mechanisms for maintaining the daily territorial status quo, such as scent marking. Nevertheless, in cases where an important food source lies near the border of two neighbouring territories, the territorial aggression can escalate: on one such border I witnessed over 46 clashes during a two-month period. While most of my evidence on territoriality comes from only three study areas, my more fragmentary observations elsewhere, together with those of most other studies, support their generality. Territoriality within the fox population has important consequences for any control scheme that involves killing foxes (such as that operative in France in recent years). This point can best be explained by reference to studies done on other animals, in particular an elegant series of field experiments done by John Krebs of Oxford University.

Krebs has been studying the behavioural ecology of great tits in the Oxfordshire woodland. The great tits are strictly territorial, forming pairs that defend their particular patch against all comers. By walking repeatedly around his study area and plotting the course of all observations on a map (each bird was individually recognisable by means of a coloured leg ring), Krebs was able to draw a map depicting the exact boundaries between territories holding eight pairs of great tits. At the same time he tape-recorded the individual calls of the birds concerned.

On a particular morning in February he removed all the resident birds from their territories. In some territories (called 'experimental') he replaced the birds with loud-speakers that played the recorded songs of the original residents at appropriate intervals, while in the other territories (called 'controls') the speakers played some irrelevant noise during the same time. The loud-speakers began at 2.00 p.m. on the chosen day and Krebs watched the empty territories during all the daylight hours until midday two days later. By then all the vacant territories had been refilled and eight new pairs of great tits were in residence. Interestingly, all the control territories were completely filled within eight daylight hours; some of the new owners were already singing their ownership within six hours. The 'experimental' territories took slightly longer to fill, demonstrating the role of song in proclaiming ownership — a role that might well be played by scent in foxes. The interesting question is where did the new occupants come from? and the answer was twofold: some came from neighbouring hedgerows where they maintained territories but where the habitat is known to be less appropriate (suboptimal) for the bird; others came from a floating population of non-residents that moves through the wood, passing through occupied territories in much the same way as the dispersing foxes described above.

I have chosen the example of the great tits to illustrate the point as it is perhaps the most complete and refined study to date, but the same trends have been shown for many other species. The implications are clear for foxes — that the death of territory holders may be compensated for almost at once by an influx of new animals from the 'sink', leaving the overall situation little different, but having stimulated considerable local movement. The parallel between Krebs's experiments and the efforts of the French authorities to stem the westward tide of rabies by mass slaughter of foxes along a belt, one-hundred kilometres wide, across the country, is striking and one might be tempted to speculate that the result was a vacuum effect, drawing foxes into vacant ranges. However, both Lloyd and Jensen, a Danish biologist, have doubts on the speed with which foxes do recolonize cleared areas and clearly this will vary with the size of the area concerned and probably from one season to the next. Amongst resident foxes the death of one resident can cause unusual movement of its neighbours. I have found vixens making temporary excursions into the range of a neighbour poisoned the previous night and have even seen a vixen trespass at a feeding site within the territory of another that was absent having had cubs only hours before. It is clear that the social behaviour of both tits and foxes is complex and finely tuned and that both can respond almost astonishingly quickly to changes. A further consequence of killing territory holders that has already been demonstrated for animals as diverse as sticklebacks, blackbirds, and monkeys is that during stimulation of activity the newcomers may pack in more tightly than their predecessors resulting in a higher population density than before. Furthermore, there may be qualitative changes in the relationship between new and old residents: Bertram has demonstrated the so-called 'dear enemy' phenomenon amongst mynah birds whereby residents are familiar with the individual voices of their neighbours and pay them little heed as long as the status quo is maintained. However, as soon as a stranger's voice is heard, the newcomer may provoke vigorous aggression. Where the population has a rapid turnover the frequency of aggressive inter-territorial contact might escalate between unfamiliar neighbours who do not 'know the ropes'. The speed and pattern with which the 'sink' of non-resident foxes can fill empty slots is at present under study.

There is yet a further complication: the territories that I have been describing for foxes are occupied by not one nor even a pair of adults, but rather by a group. In areas where the foxes are unmolested by man, which are, admittedly, few and far between, there are family groups numbering up to six animals, including one dog fox together with several vixens. The factors influencing the size of these groups are not yet fully understood but they probably involve an interplay between food, predation pressure, and social mechanisms, of which the latter may yet prove to be the most important.

It is interesting to note that the Nature Conservancy biologists analysing the foxes killed in Scotland since 1948 have recently recorded a change in the ratio of adults to cubs in favour of adults. They conclude that this indicates either a lower survival rate of cubs or a reduced reproductive rate amongst the vixens. This can be considered in conjunction with other data such as that collected in Sweden where markedly different birth rates in different habitat types seemed partially explicable by the numbers of 'barren' vixens present in any one area which varies between the enormous limits of 35 per cent and 74 per cent.

On the basis of the productivity of the wild vixens within my stable family groups, together with preliminary results from a long term study of captive foxes, the notion that some social factor influences vixen productivity cannot be dismissed. It is perhaps worth considering, in this context, the known behaviour of the wolf, a related carnivore. Wolves live in packs, the size of which seems to be largely determined by the size of their principal prey species within a given area. In a pack there may be several dogs and bitches together with a number of young. During any one year it is customary for only one bitch, normally the so-called alpha or dominant bitch, to rear cubs. The entire reproductive effort of the pack is then invested in her offspring. It is interesting to speculate that, if such a mechanism operated in foxes, then the death of the reproductive vixen (who would probably be the most vulnerable to man's attention) might simply release other vixens from a suppressive influence that had previously inhibited their breeding. There would, again, be only a limited long term effect on the population.

Another suggestion, advanced, amongst others, by Schofield, is that the average litter size increases when the population is cut by intensive control. Again, much more work is needed before this hypothesis can be adequately tested, but it is worth noting that a study done in Ohio by Phillips demonstrated a ratio of 2·56 cubs to every one adult in an area with little control, but of 5·59 cubs per adult in an area with severe control. Whatever the mechanism may be by which this compensation is achieved, it does mean that any control is, to an extent, counter-balanced by the animal's reaction to it.

The commonly held notion of the fox as a solitary animal is, to me, unrealistic. Even if in some areas the social system is disrupted by human pressure, the species clearly has the capacity to live in complex and highly integrated social groups. The fact that the members of these groups do not engage in any conspicuous activity involving co-operating (such as hunting of big prey, as do members of wolf packs) does not make them 'unsocial', but rather it means that we have to search for other functions for their social organization. The death of a fox, whether as a victim of rabies or of some control scheme designed to halt the disease, will have a different effect on the remaining foxes depending on whether the deceased was a territory holder or not, a dog or a vixen, a senior or junior member of the group, or whether it is summer or winter. Clearly the epidemiologist faces a complex problem, and it is hardly surprising that steps to halt the disease have met with such varied success.

Through the course of history rabies has come and gone, indeed in Europe between 1803 and 1925 there were seven major fox epizooties. The present threat is of a new wave of the disease that began its west-ward course from Poland in 1939, reaching the west bank of the Elbe in 1950, and the Rhine by 1960. By 1967 it had entered Belgium and Luxembourg and penetrated France in 1968. In spite of expansive assassination schemes launched against foxes the disease spread unerringly westward and by the end of March 1976 it threatened Chantilly, the racehorse centre twenty-five miles from Paris. Fearing for the seventy million pounds worth of racehorses stabled there, the Chantilly authorities hired fifteen men to gas fox earths with Zyklon B (the same product employed in Auschwitz). It is the forward march of rabies to the French coast and thence towards the British Isles that has given rise to the present scare, although the risk must always have been substantial in recent years since pets have been smuggled into Britain from inland France and, indeed, elsewhere in Europe.

Since rabies appears to have come and gone repeatedly, we must ask what precipitates an outbreak. The build-up of a rabies epizooty often seems to be associated with increases in the density of fox (or other vector) populations and it is suggested that such an increase, due to the lack of predation on foxes during the Second World War, enhanced the spread of the present epizooty. This generalization seems particularly true for outbreaks in the far north amongst Arctic foxes, the last of which was between 1950 and 1953 in the Canadian Arctic. During these years peak Arctic fox numbers were recorded. Similarly, a major outbreak in Nenet, in the Northern U.S.S.R., coincided with an apparent increase in Arctic fox numbers, together with a substantial fox migration. The Russian scientist describing this latter outbreak noted significant differences in the extent to which different sections of the fox population were infected. For instance, young foxes and males of all ages were infected to twice the extent of females. This difference might relate to the observations that males of all ages and young foxes (certainly of the red fox species) are more likely to be involved in dispersal movements and hence in ensuing aggressive encounters, with other foxes on whose territory they trespass. This may also have some bearing on the markedly seasonal nature of the disease in Russia where it is only present from November to March. In much of Europe there is an annual peak in late winter to March. This is just over a month after the time when vixens are in oestrous and may be the interval required during which symptoms could develop after the peak of social contact around mating. The incidence of rabid foxes is thus when the fox population is at its lowest, but when certain types of social interaction and movement are at a peak.

Another suggestion is that the rabies virus can lie dormant in a host, only to re-emerge at times of 'stress' (which may also be times of high population density or social interaction). This idea stems partially from the discovery that in some areas 3 per cent of the foxes possess rabies neutralizing antibodies, suggesting that they have survived the disease and might possibly act as carriers. Evidence suggests that female skunks may show a reactivation of latent rabies virus due to the stress of rearing young. There has also been an experimental demonstration of the reactivation of a latent infection of rabies amongst guinea pigs when they were kept in overcrowded and hence 'stressed' conditions (See Chapter 1).

The 'carrier' hypothesis has also been confirmed in bats in the United States. There it has been demonstrated that the rabies virus can be stored in the bats' brown fat. In the breeding season the fat is metabolized under the physiological stress of breeding and the virus is passed on to juveniles. The age and sex classes shown to be prone to the infection amongst Russian Arctic foxes might be considered to be those under most stress. Indeed, I have analysed the fat content of dispersing dog foxes during the winter in the United Kingdom, and it is clear that they often have little left by way of reserves. The outbreak of an epizooty in other vectors, such as skunks, is also thought to tie up with peak years in population density and they are thought to be able to act as carriers of the disease during intervening years.

Skunks, incidentally, are now more important vectors for the American rabies epizooty than foxes; they are particularly dangerous since they may secrete rabies virus through their salivary glands for as long as eighteen days before death. This clearly gives them ample opportunity to infect others (which is particularly significant as they may live in communal dens) in comparison with the three to four-day infective period which is quoted as the norm for the fox. Indeed the build-up of virus in the fox's saliva and the duration of its infective period depends largely on the original quantity of infecting virus. Without mild infections, which result from relatively minor wounds and take a long time to run their course, the infected foxes would probably die so quickly that they would have little opportunity for passing on the infection. In such circumstances, reservoirs, such as the skunk, could be crucial to the survival of the virus. Recently the raccoon has joined the forward line of American rabies vectors, particularly around Florida. Evidence suggests that the disease does, indeed, lie latent in the raccoon and that the epizootic outbreaks are associated with some stress factor in the population which causes the latent virus to emerge.

The situation in the United States, with a variety of different vectors each with a different behavioural ecology and epidemiology, presents a far more complex problem than that in Europe. (See Chapter 1.) It has been suggested that weasels, stoats or martens might act as a reservoir for the disease in Europe (playing the role of the skunk by infecting foxes every time the disease looked like fading out) but no evidence has been found to verify this, although the number of these small carnivores dying from the disease is probably underestimated because of the low probability of noticing them.

By whatever means an epizootic wave begins, once it has started it can spread quite rapidly. Whether or not it spreads amongst the vector population is widely assumed to depend on the population density of the vector and hence the opportunity for social contact and infection (and perhaps the level of stress). In 1948 H.T. Gier suggested that a fox density of two per square mile would support an epizooty. This seems to be confirmed since three per square mile supported an outbreak in New York while one per square mile failed to do so. In France rabies spreads in areas where the estimated fox population is four per square mile. However, these population figures are at best only estimates since making a realistic census of fox numbers requires long and careful observation of one small area, and has rarely been attempted. Nevertheless, an American rabies authority, Winkler, has performed the following simple calculation: 'Assuming that a fox's territory extends two miles (Sargeant 1972), and allowing thirty days between exposure and subsequent virus shedding, the expected rate of movement in a hypothetical population would be twenty-four miles (thirty-eight km) per year.'

Winkler is fully aware of, and carefully states, the limitations of such simplistic calculations. Nevertheless, this shows the way in which we can extrapolate from range-size data and the estimate does fall within the estimated spread of epidemic fronts for both Europe and the United States of between thirty and sixty kilometres per year. In fact the quoted average figure of two miles (Sargeant states one to three) related to an area of two square miles. This, in a circular range, would be equivalent to a diameter of 2553 metres and a potential spread of the disease of 30·6 km (19·2 miles) per year. Of course animal home ranges are normally very irregular shapes and, if anything, might corres-pond more closely to elipses than circles. However, we can assume a circle for this sort of rough calculation since we have seen that territory size varies greatly. It is interesting to see what difference is made to these estimates of the rate of spread of rabies by substituting other values for the territory diameter.

The smallest ranges I have found were less than thirty hectares. These ranges were, of course, an irregular shape, but if the kinks were ironed out and they were made circular they would have a diameter of about 618 metres. Substituting this value in Winkler's calculation (instead of two miles), the disease would spread at approximately 7·4 km (4·6 miles) per year. At the other extreme are my ranges of over 1300 hectares which would be equivalent to circular ranges of diameter of 4068 metres. Using this value, the disease might spread at 48·8 km (30 miles) per year. The same simple calculation can be applied to the quoted figure of four foxes per square mile, or 256 hectares, in France: the social organisation of these four foxes will influence their potential contribution to the spread of the disease. For instance, if they consist of two pairs occupying territories of 128 hectares (half a square mile) each, then (using the thirty-day interval) the disease would spread through 15·3 km (9·5 miles) per year. If they are arranged in a group of four foxes in one territory of 256 hectares (and neglecting the effect of group size on the probability of infection) the potential spread would be a third as far again, 21·7 km (13·5 miles) per year. All these figures fall short of the maximum recorded annual spread and it is interesting to ask what territory size would be required to achieve this (assuming only territory holders are involved, as in Winkler's calculation). To achieve a spread of between 30 and 60 km (18·6 and 37·2 miles) per year would require ranges of diameter 2500 to 5000 metres (1·6 to 3·1 miles). Of course in reality these figures would require correction for the way interaction frequency changed as a function of home range size.

It seems improbable that resident foxes are maintaining sufficiently large territories to give rise to the maximum annual spread and so two possibilities must be investigated. First, that another social category, such as itinerant or dispersing foxes, is responsible for the transmission, or, second, that the behaviour of non-rabid foxes is different from that of rabid foxes. It is worth noting that from ear-tagging studies by Jensen, we know that of young Danish foxes (less than one year old) 80 per cent of the males and 31 per cent of the females disperse for a straightline distance of over five km (3·1 miles). This is to say that if they were infected, approximately 55 per cent of young foxes in Denmark would travel far enough to spread the disease at the fastest observed annual rate of sixty km (37·2 miles) per year. Incidentally, using the same data, 38 per cent of the cubs might travel more than fifteen km (19·3 miles) which might potentially spread the disease at 180 km (111·8 miles) per year and why this does not happen is not clear. The second possibility is of changes in the behaviour of a rabid fox and in reactions to it, but little is known about this. Winkler has twice observed a healthy fox in a cage with a rabid one: on one occasion the healthy animal shied away from the sick one, while in the second it licked its saliva. In neither case did the rabid fox attack the non-rabid fox. Foxes do not seem to exhibit the maniacal symptoms associated with furiously rabid dogs. Like Winkler, I use these calculations not in a pretence that they are realistic, but rather to stress the sort of factors that might influence the spread of rabies through the fox population.

From the foregoing observations one can begin to imagine how many foxes might have to be destroyed if we act on the prevalent notion that destroying foxes is the way to stem the tide of rabies. Intensive 'population reduction' schemes have been widely employed but most people in this country have no idea of the actual scale of some of these operations (few realize that pest control officials already kill over one thousand foxes per year in Bromley): the most dramatic example that has been credited with success was an effort in 1952 to stop the southerly spread of rabies through the province of Alberta. One hundred and eighty trappers were employed to work 48·3 km (30 miles) of trapline each; they used 6000 cyanide capsules, and 429 000 strychnine cubes. During an eighteen-month period the *minimum* total kill numbered 50 000 foxes, 35 000 coyotes, 4300 wolves, 7500 lynx, 1850 bears, 500 skunks, 64 cougar, 1 wolverine and 4 badgers. The scheme was supported by an extension programme in which farmers were supplied with 75 000 cyanide shells and 163 000 strychnine pellets (killing an estimated 60 000 to 80 000 coyotes).

The Alberta project does not stand alone: in an effort to stamp out rabies in Mexico, cubes of horse meat containing sodium mono-fluoroacetate poison were placed over 15 540 square km (6000 square miles), claiming an estimated 18 000 wolves, coyotes, foxes, and skunks on the Mexican mainland, together with 10 000 more on the peninsula of Baja California. Coyotes were said to be exterminated over an area of 12 800 square km (5000 square miles). As might be expected, such schemes are expensive and it was estimated that each fox killed during a Tennessee scheme cost 208 dollars. Apart from the grotesque inhumanity of these methods, there are again predictable backlashes: the removal of predators frequently has a profound effect on the population stability of their prey species. In Alberta numbers of deer and moose escalated after the slaughter of carnivores, resulting in serious overgrazing and consequent long term damage to the range, reducing its capacity to maintain big game herds.

One wonders that man's ingenuity cannot contrive some more elegant answer than blanket assassination schemes, but these can be judged fairly only on the basis of answers to two questions: first, do they work? and second, is there an alternative that works equally well? The answers, of course, are equivocal — some schemes have apparently succeeded, for instance, the Alberta one, together with those in Denmark, parts of Germany (although only to a limited extent), while the French and Swiss have failed. Other outbreaks have seemingly died out in the absence of any control and we cannot guess what would have happened in those areas where control was exerted if they had been left alone. At least part of the answer to why some population reduction schemes have succeeded and others have not must lie in the habitat type involved and the resulting ease or difficulty involved in trapping. Even more important, I believe, may be differences in the behavioural ecology of the fox in different areas, consequent largely upon the sort of differences in diet discussed earlier.

A 75 per cent reduction in fox population size is often quoted as the minimum that will achieve any long-lasting (more than one generation) effect (although this must vary depending on population density, immigration/emigration rates etc.). Only highly experienced local trappers could even guess at the feasibility in practical terms of achieving this target. Thus, in the past, the decision on what to do has been difficult and it is too easy to be critical of failure in retrospect. Nevertheless, one can quote Parks who noted that post-epizooty trapping was ineffective except from the public relations viewpoint. That, in my view, is not a good enough reason for doing it! Today we have the background knowledge and equipment for tackling the problem in a more scientific way, initiating studies in advance of the outbreak and also monitoring the detailed response of foxes (or other vectors) affected by attempted control schemes. Future contingency plans should be biologically appropriate to a given time and place. This is being done in several European countries, including Holland. A project is just beginning in the Italian Alps with which I am involved. The Alps form an important physical barrier between Italy, which is free from rabies, and her infected neighbours. There is considerable public concern, exacerbated by alarmist reports, that the disease may cross in foxes travelling through the high passes. We are currently trying to radio-collar foxes on both the French and Italian sides to discover whether the behaviour and ecology of the fox precludes or admits this risk, and to investigate the possibility of effective control measures, in particular vaccination (see below and Chapter 7). Preliminary observations suggest that, in such inhospitable country, 'population reduction' schemes would be so impractical as to be valueless. The emphasis placed by the Italians (under the guidance of Professor Biocca) on biological realism is encouraging and is perhaps in contrast to another Italian proposal, endorsed this year, to attempt to exterminate foxes from a thrity-kilometre wide strip across the mountains and hence to prevent the possible spread of rabies from Switzerland. This will be done with strychnine baits (because trapping is judged impractical in alpine terrain) and will presumably affect other predators ranging from martens to golden eagles in a previously unmolested part of Europe. It may work, but if so, will it be through luck or judgement?

As to alternatives: until recently these have not existed, even as concepts, and even now they remain in their infancy. In my view the most exciting idea is one originating amongst such American virologists as Baer and Winkler, stemming from original observations by Remlinger in 1959. Noting the widespread failure of population reduction, they have begun investigating the possibility of vaccinating vectors, including foxes, in the field. To date their work has been confined to the laboratory, studying the immunological problems such as the most appropriate methods and sites of innoculation. They have discovered that food containing vaccine placed directly in the stomach has no effect, but the same food *eaten* by the fox gave 78 per cent of the foxes immunity. Now they have localised the portal of entry of the vaccine as the pharyngeal mucosa. Other workers have experimented with freeze-dried vaccine and obtained promising results (thirteen out of sixteen foxes that had eaten the vaccine lived while eleven out of fourteen unvaccinated foxes died when both groups were challenged with the live virus). One serious complication is that a vaccine strong enough to give immunity to the fox might actually cause the disease if eaten by another species and this happens where, for instance, the cotton rat is given a fox dose.

Even when the complications of the technique have been fully resolved the next main problem will be how to use it. Field trials involving the capture, vaccination, and release of wild foxes are beginning in Germany and Switzerland. However, capture is difficult and expensive. Ways must be found of getting the foxes to vaccinate themselves, perhaps by eating treated baits. Work is beginning on this in Canada and my own project will also focus on these practical problems. One of the first questions to be asked is how the distribution and number of baits should be organized to ensure sufficient foxes receive the vaccination. The answer will be different depending on the local fox ecology. Clearly we will need to know even more about the factors affecting territory size and ranging behaviour to solve this.

Other suggestions for control include the use of a gametocide, a drug fed to the foxes in bait that would destroy their reproductive capacity. While this idea seems recently to have fallen from fashion, it would have the advantages of (a) not creating a vacuum effect, and (b) permitting the continued operation of any social suppression on reproduction that may exist in stable fox communities.

The discussion so far has centred on situations where rabies is already established. With the exception of the outbreak between 1919 and 1922 (see Chapter 1) we have not had rabies in Britain since 1903. Before that it was rife amongst the canine population. Apparently rabies was not present in our foxes, although it plagued the packs of hounds that hunted them in the nineteenth century. Why this was so is not known. The fox population may well have been much smaller during the nineteenth century than it is today, but why it did not contract rabies thereafter is a mystery. Whatever the reason, there is no need for complacency since the present widespread distribution of foxes throughout Britain, and the close proximity between our towns and rural land which are bridged by the suburban fox and cat populations, all spell potential disaster *if* the disease ever became established in this country.

Indeed, our position is particularly hazardous concerning domestic animals too, with our small island harbouring over six million dogs and the same number of cats. Gwyn Lloyd discusses in detail in Chapter 6 contingency plans in the event of rabies getting into our wildlife, and I shall only mention that one idea is to hit the infected animals rapidly within an area of radius 22 km (14 miles) using up to 7900 poisoned baits. Of course a circle of radius 22 kilometres (area 152 053 hectares, 608 square miles) may contain vastly different numbers of foxes depending on the habitat: using my *extreme* figures for territory size (and ignoring itinerant foxes) this circle could contain between 116 and 5068 territories, or using the probably more general territory size of 250 hectares (1 square mile) it would contain 608 territories. Each territory, as we have seen, may contain several foxes. The calculated risk is that against these odds the critical animal might be missed and that the death of others will increase local movement and enhance the spread of the disease. The alternative — doing nothing and allowing the disease to take a hold – is completely untenable. We can only hope that through public awareness, and vigilance at our ports the situation will not arise. In the meantime it should be clear from the discussion above that any attempt to reduce the fox population now in anticipation of a possible outbreak that may never happen, would be unwarranted and pointless. Some of the new research initiated throughout the world as a consequence of the rabies problem seems to me indicative of a most heartening and necessary change in the relationship between man and his environment; the fruits of a marriage between practical problems and academic pursuits may be a biologically integrated approach to wildlife management.

The rabies issue is one of many complicated problems of wildlife management facing the world today. As it comes within our reach to study and understand the workings of nature, it is imperative that we use this knowledge in ways that allow us to achieve the desired end with minimum disturbance to the ecological balance we have already distorted so badly. This may sometimes require a new relationship between western man and his environment: one frequently reads of fox population reduction schemes where, acknowledging the enormous potential for adverse side effects on other species and the ecosystem in general, officials decided it was, nevertheless, necessary to use poison as the control method because it was the 'cheapest' . . . Cheapest on what scale of values?

6

Wildlife rabies: prospects for Britain

H. G. LLOYD

Since Britain is an island, it should be possible to keep rabies out. In present circumstances any introduction of the disease would be the result of deliberate or unintentional evasion of quarantine, or of fortuitous transport of infected mammals as stowaways by sea or by air. The probability of such events cannot be assessed but as wildlife rabies advances through France and, before long, possibly Spain, it can only increase. The natural spread of rabies from Europe to Britain by winged animals is not at present an important threat, since very few birds and bats are implicated in rabies outbreaks in Europe. Thus, unless there is a dramatic change in the ecology of rabies and its pattern of spread, the main threat is posed by international traffic.

As indicated by Kaplan in the first chapter, the reservoir of rabies in Europe is the wild mammal population, and its occurrence in domestic animals is an over-spill from the disease in wild mammals. Outbreaks in dogs and cats in developed countries can be successfully contained by vaccination, restraint, confinement, or elimination of infected animals. Widespread self-perpetuating outbreaks in dogs and cats are prevented by such measures. Wild mammals cannot be restrained. It may be difficult, and it is certainly aesthetically and biologically undesirable, to eliminate them; and vaccination of wild life, though experimentally successful in Europe and North America for some species, is a recent innovation not yet proved by extensive field trials.

The inability to control rabies in wild mammals is responsible for the inexorable advance of rabies westward from Eastern Europe since about 1940. In Western Europe the ubiquitous red fox is the main vector of the disease. European research workers consider that in the absence of the fox, other wild species singly or collectively could not maintain the disease overtly. Some consider that badgers might in some localities be an exception, and possibly also the raccoon dog (*Nyctereutes procyonoides*), an asiatic alien spreading westward from Eastern Europe.

Carnivores are clearly implicated as the most important vectors of rabies. In North America the pattern of wildlife rabies is different and more complex from that in Europe since it enjoys a richer carnivore fauna. The species mostly implicated are the red and grey foxes, two species of skunks, badgers and raccoons, and, in the north, wolves and arctic foxes. In addition, in the southern parts of Canada, the U.S., Central America, and much of South America, rabies is present in bats.

Because wild carnivores include the most potent rabies vectors, it is reasonable to suppose that the greatest threat in Britain would be from the fox. For this reason the Pest Infestation Control Laboratory of the Ministry of Agriculture, Fisheries, and Food has investigated those aspects of the ecology and behaviour of foxes which are pertinent to the spread of rabies and the control of foxes. European experience of wildlife rabies is of considerable help in understanding problems that would arise in Britain in the event of an outbreak of the disease in wild mammals. In Europe rabies in any area is usually first advertized by its occurrence in foxes. Europeans estimate that infected fox populations are reduced by between 20 per cent and 60 per cent by the disease. This variable mortality is probably a reflection of differing fox population densities and, in turn, of habitats. The fox is a nonspecific predator on a fairly wide range of small animals, a scavenger and a feeder on fruit, and occasionally vegetables; an opportunistic feeder that thrives best in fragmented habitats offering a wide variety of food and cover.

Continental workers estimate that densities higher than one adult or sub-adult fox per square km will successfully sustain an outbreak of rabies whereas one fox per 5 square km will not. The precise threshold where the shift would occur is not known, nor would it be entirely realistic to define the threshold, since foxes may not be evenly dispersed even throughout a large area, whatever the overall density. The occurrence of rabies in foxes, though not seasonal, shows a distinct seasonal peak in numbers infected in late autumn and winter, a time of year when the fox population is least sedentary and most unsettled in its behaviour. The rate of spread of rabies into uninfected areas varies from 20 to 60 km a year. This variability is again probably a reflection of the effects of differing densities and habitats. In urban areas the rate of spread tends to be low. In the wake of the advancing front of the disease sporadic and intermittent outbreaks occur in a zone 50 to 80 km deep for many months, usually followed by another outbreak 3 to 4 years later, among those groups which have increased in numbers. Such outbreaks may recur subsequently with the same order of periodicity. A similar periodicity was first reported among foxes in Canada.

The incubation period, that is the period between infection and (approximately) the onset of rabies symptoms, varies so far as is known from about 15 to 40 days. A rabid fox loses its natural timidity and shows no fear of man or his domestic animals. It does not go out of its way to attack an intruder but will unhesitatingly do so if one gets in its way.

North American rabid foxes have been found with porcupine quills embedded in their faces — a testimony to their abnormal behaviour in attacking an animal they normally shun. The period of fearlessness when rabies can be transmitted by bite lasts some 4 to 7 days, before death supervenes. Unlike many rabid dogs there does not seem to be a general tendency to retreat to dark, quiet places. Foxes are highly susceptible to a rabid bite. They are often known to transmit the disease to dogs but there is no direct evidence of domestic animals infecting wild mammals. This might occur, of course, but it is effectively masked by the prevalence of the disease in wild mammals. This was, however, almost certainly the route of transmission to wild mammals on the islands of Sicily and Corsica and, earlier, in France in 1925 (the disease was successfully eliminated in foxes and badgers in 1928).

The methods of anti-rabies fox control which have been used on the continent to try and eliminate infected animals and reduce population densities of foxes so that rabies cannot spread further, are shooting, gassing and poisoning. With the single exception of Denmark none in the long term has succeeded in attaining the objectives. Rabies is still present in foxes in Poland now, some 36 years since its first appearance there. It is estimated that at the present rate of spread France will be infected throughout by 1990. If wildlife rabies persists in France, Germany, and the other countries nearest to Britain for as long as it has in Poland the probability of a rabid domestic animal being introduced to Britain will increase — in the absence of rabies alarms — as the general public become inured to its presence across the water, and perhaps as methods of prophylaxis and treatment of human patients improve and become known. Doubtless sooner or later a rabid mammal will be introduced by one avenue or another, but this is as speculative as is an appraisal of the probability of wildlife becoming infected. Account cannot be taken of all eventualities but the most predictable situation is direct infection of wildlife by dogs and cats. The chances of a major widespread outbreak among dogs and cats from a single introduction seem to be remote in view of the wide powers that the State Veterinary Service have in this context.

A more realistic situation would be a small number of dogs or cats becoming infected in a circumscribed area. There are many examples of foxes and dogs — even foxes and cats — forming friendly associations, most commonly in suburban areas. Usually however, there is little direct physical contact between non-working household pets and foxes. A paralytic or semi-paralytic rabid dog may attract the attention of a fox but the fox is unlikely to approach closely until the dog clearly poses no threat. Remains of dogs, probably road casualties, have been found at suburban cubbing den sites testifying to the fox's scavenging habits. Clearly there are situations where foxes could encounter a rabid dog − orphaned cubs, friendly foxes, and chance encounters − but the possibility seems to be very small if only one dog or a few dogs are involved. The short period that the dog is infective and can effectively transmit the virus by bite, and its abnormal behaviour tend to reduce the probability of encounters with adult foxes.

The cat, however, poses a somewhat greater threat of transmission to wildlife, since there is evidence that foxes do occasionally attack and kill cats. Conversely, and interestingly, observers have reported cats behaving antagonistically towards foxes! Certainly foxes seem to show less regard to the close proximity of cats than of dogs, though this may simply be a reflection of the fox's ability to discriminate visually between dogs and cats but not between cats and other similarly-sized potential prey. The fox's eye is designed for good visual acuity but its brain is not capable of discriminating immobile shapes that it sees − as many countrymen well know. At long range, the pattern of movement of an animal will provide more information to an experienced fox than its shape. Gamekeepers assert that in gin-trapping days one of the most effective baits or lures for a fox was a dead cat. Whether or not this be true the cat does indeed figure fairly frequently in the diet of fox cubs. Many, if not all, of these cats might be the product of local scavenging upon road casualties, which could put foxes at risk since it is hypothetically possible for a fox to become infected by eating a freshly dead rabid cat, or any other infected species. The opportunistic propensities of foxes to exploit situations (as in the fables) could well put a normally cat-fearing fox at risk when investigating a vulnerable cat in the late stages of the disease. The probability of any such events is dependent upon a variety of circumstances but whilst the risk is small it could occur as it has done in Sicily and Corsica.

Clearly the risk increases directly with the number of domestic animals infected and, for the reasons given, would probably be greater with cats than with dogs. The risk of park deer becoming infected by dogs would probably be much greater than foxes; but the disease tends to be a dead-end in deer. The possibility of transmission of the disease from domestic to wild carnivores other than foxes seems to be small; for example it seems most improbable that a rabid dog would seek a dark retreat in a badger set, though if it did the likelihood of transmission would be high, since the badger would almost certainly survive the physical encounter. Of intermediaries bridging infection from dog to fox, the impregnable hedgehog (and the porcupine in North America) would probably be the most likely candidate.

Fortuitous introductions of rabid animals could quickly give rise to serious circumstances especially if the disease were transmitted to dogs or cats, since the time and origin of the outbreak would probably not be known. The most likely stowaway would be a rodent or a small carnivore and, among domestic animals, most probably the cat. One of the best safeguards against this would be the discouragement or removal of stray dogs and cats at docks, airports, and marinas, but container cargo is another possible route of entry and this may be discharged anywhere.

Anti-rabies control in foxes in Britain, whether on a large or small scale, presents problems less daunting than on the Continent. Today, about one-sixth of the area of France is infected, and attempts to prevent further spread along the frontal zone some 700 km long, let alone eliminate the disease behind the advancing front, would be an enormously complex and costly operation. In Britain, the aim would be the elimination of all infected foxes as quickly as possible to prevent further spread. Action would be required to reduce fox numbers to very low levels within prescribed areas in order to ensure the best probability of removing all infected animals — drastic action which would be justified by the penalties of failure.

Confirmation of the disease in a wild fox would initiate swift action. Fortunately, the comparatively long incubation period, the short infective period, and the obviously unusual behaviour of rabid foxes (which would advertize their condition) reduce the risk of rapid dissemination of the disease by a single animal. But the high mobility of foxes tends to offset this, and would require action to be taken over a much larger area than in the immediate vicinity of the location of an infected animal. Knowledge of the biology of foxes is required to determine the size of the area over which action would be required, the methods to be used, and whether or not these two features would need to be varied according to time and place. The size of the area would be determined not so much by the movements of rabid foxes (which, judging from European experience, are not large) but by the normal movements of healthy but infected foxes between the time of infection and the time when they are capable of transmitting the infection.

The normal movements of foxes are their dispersal from one home area to another and their ranging movements within the area in which they live. In autumn juvenile foxes tend to move away from their 'family group' areas, where they were born and reared, to settle elsewhere. Such dispersal movements are more pronounced among male foxes, and in hill and lowland areas in Mid-Wales average 14 km (8·5 miles). Some foxes barely shift from their places of birth; others move up to 50 km (30 miles). Ten per cent of juvenile males move more than 20 km (12 miles). Juvenile vixens are less adventurous, moving on average 2·5 km (1·5 miles), though a few move 15 to 25 km (10 to 15 miles). This information is based on the tagging of over 400 cubs since 1965. In West Wales 108 tagged cubs revealed smaller dispersal movements: an average of 4·8 km (2·9 miles) for males and 2 km (1·2 miles) for females. Similarly obtained data for urban areas suggest that dispersal movements are of an order rather similar to those by West Wales. Clearly, there is much variation; more information is required for different rural and urban habitats and, if possible, to determine cause and effect relationships. The annual rate of spread of rabies in Europe (20 to 60 km per year) indicates an overall pattern of steady though seasonal advancement into rabies-free areas rather than outbreaks well ahead of the advancing front followed by an infilling of the intermediate rabies-free areas. The seasonal and annual rates of spread are not inconsistent with the average dispersal distances described in Mid-Wales and suggest, where distances covered are small, as in West Wales, that the abnormal movements of rabid foxes exceed the small dispersal distances of foxes in similar habitats in Europe.

Recapturing foxes tagged as adults indicates that very few long-range movements occur after a fox has settled in a new area during its first year of adult life. Foxes have been recovered as long as 5 years later in the same den in which they were originally caught and tagged. Settled foxes clearly do not move far, but little can be learned about the areas over which settled tagged foxes range (their home ranges) without a more sophisticated technique. The attachment of radio transmitters to foxes and the monitoring of their movements by radio telemetry has provided a considerable insight into dispersal and home range behaviour. The movement of 34 juvenile male foxes fitted with radio transmitters has been observed during dispersal. No generalized pattern of behaviour has emerged. However, evidence obtained in this way in North America suggests that male juveniles may suddenly disperse over quite long distances with little deviation from the original direction of departure from its family group range. This has been observed in Wales, but more usually the foxes travel comparatively short distances of less than 3·3 km (2 miles) per night, in a different direction each night, and often return to their point of origin after several days' absence. Such forays may be followed by comparatively sedentary behaviour before another journey is undertaken — usually in the direction of one of the areas previously visited. Dispersal may take a few days but more usually the period of unsettled behaviour may last a few weeks. The greatest recorded point-to-point dispersal movement undertaken in one night was 13·3 km (8 miles).

Dispersal is not synchronous throughout the juvenile male component of the population — some foxes are unsettled from October, others disperse over a shorter period in December — but the peak period is December to early January. Settled adult foxes or dispersed juveniles which have forged or otherwise acquired a range in their new area in January will move away from their range when hunted or when disturbed by shooting parties, but they will return to it after dark. Dispersing juvenile males, or males which have made reconnaissance movements but have not moved away from their family group range, behave similarly when disturbed by hunting and shooting but, unlike the others, may not return to the area where they were hunted. Thus, in some circumstances, dispersal can be precipitated by human interference. Foxes are relentlessly pursued in the primarily sheep-rearing areas of Mid-Wales and it may well be that man's anti-fox activities are in some measure responsible for the large-scale dispersal movements compared with those of foxes living in comparative peace in West Wales. The killing of vixens between December and February may also influence the behaviour of males in their immediate vicinity; and it probably has more effect on the movements of juveniles which have only a slender attachment to a newly acquired area, than on those of adult dogs with a long-standing attachment.

A few juvenile dog foxes continue to be itinerant even in May. These may be some of the 17 per cent of surplus males in the population (the sex ratio of over 15 000 foxes examined in Wales was 54 per cent male).

Dispersal of juvenile vixens has not been so well studied, but they tend to conform to a generalized pattern of a slight shift in early winter. Some, however, move unaccountably after they have become pregnant (the period of mating in such foxes is calculated from the time of birth of their cubs). Vixens of any age which fail to breed (22·5 per cent in Wales in some years) do not appear to behave differently in their movements from other vixens. Irrespective of the stimulus to disperse and the distances dispersed there is considerable social contact between foxes in autumn and winter; consequently this would be the period when rabies would spread readily, most swiftly, and widely.

Fox home range behaviour and range size are less important to the rapid spread of rabies but have some significance for the control of foxes. Ranges seem mostly to be overlapping, non-exclusive and of variable size ranging from less than 40 hectares (c. 100 acres) to 1500 hectares (6 square miles). Within these there may be small areas which are exclusive, as in the vicinity of cubbing dens. Ranges can be any shape, even like a string of beads with travelling routes, quickly passed through, between areas exploited for food or other resources. Contact between contiguous foxes would enable rabies to spread but not as explosively as during the dispersal period.

This would not be so, however, if settled foxes vigorously and physically defended their ranges against all intruders. Delineation of range boundaries by urination and possibly by expulsion of the secretions of the anal sacs — either on faeces or directly on to prominent objects — probably offer no more than a warning to adjacent or itinerant foxes which perhaps as a result feel less confident when they transgress. Rabid foxes would not respond in the usual way to whatever is communicated by scent marking. Movement behaviour of foxes suggests that, during the period when the spread of rabies would be potentially greatest, control would be required over an area as large as 20 km (12 miles) radius to ensure a reasonably high probability of infected foxes being contained within the prescribed zone. There should be flexibility in deciding the size of the infected zone depending upon features such as time of year, and habitat; there is no rule of thumb in determining this, it will depend on experience of foxes in the field. Swift action is essential – a predominant consideration in the choice of appropriate methods of control.

Detailed considerations of the suitability of different methods of control require further knowledge of some aspects of the behaviour of foxes. The fox is primarily a surface-dwelling animal, and tends not to seek refuge below ground during the day in areas where there is abundant surface cover. Young coniferous plantations, overgrown hedges, thickets, gorse, bracken, corn and bean fields, kale fields, disused railway lines, and boulder fields or scree provide secure cover. During inclement periods, especially when very wet, or when very hot as in the summer of 1976, foxes may seek refuge below ground even where surface cover is abundant. Vixens lie up with their cubs in daytime for the first 12 to 14 days after parturition, and at this time do not move far from the den at night. At about the time when the cubs' eyes open the vixen leaves them to lie either above ground or in another nearby earth. Cubs abandon their dens to live on the surface usually at about 8 weeks old. Dog foxes use dens intermittently during winter and early spring. Where cover is not abundant foxes lying above ground may seek refuge in dens when they are disturbed. It is possible that there is some variation in denning behaviour according to geographical location. In Mid-Wales, for example, from the time of the large increases in hill sheep numbers in the early nineteenth century, foxes have been relentlessly pursued and killed mainly by the use of terriers at dens. Elsewhere, in hunting areas, foxes tend to be killed on the surface.

Whilst the evolution of physical features by natural selection requires very long periods of time, selection for small differences in inherited behavioural traits may not; and it seems probable, in similar conditions of surface cover, that foxes in traditional hunting areas may tend to live below ground more often or seek refuge in dens with less reluctance when disturbed than in the terrier hunting areas. But this is no more than a shade of difference in behaviour in the two kinds of areas – not a complete reversal. Radio tracking studies show that on open hill in Wales foxes lying on the surface in grass or sedge will sometimes move away when intruders are as much as a mile distant – but in thick cover, or in heather, the fox will sit tight even if one is lucky enough to get within two or three yards of it; indeed, at such close quarters the fox may move off only when eye contact is made between it and the intruder.

Foxes exploit whatever cover is available in suburban areas — sometimes in earths dug in the most unlikely places. They may lie under garden sheds, on the surface in factory grounds, or in railway embankments, large gardens, or overgrown cemeteries. Suitable refuge is probably the most important factor limiting the distribution of foxes in urban areas.

Foxes are shy of strange, new objects in areas well known to them. Timidity, a suspicious nature, and unpredictable behaviour endow the fox with a talent to survive even where all hands are against it, and great skill and patience are required by those concerned in killing foxes to overcome these features. Their breeding dens may be in large earths, disused badger sets, in rabbit burrows — even single holes — and sometimes on the surface in dry ditches, under boles of trees, or in gorse and heather. If it were not for the great difficulty in locating breeding dens, foxes could well by now have been reduced to very low numbers in sheep-rearing areas.

Although shy of new objects foxes readily scavenge and will even take objects which only shortly before were discarded by a human hand. They sometimes cache food surplus to requirements, but this seems to be done less often with food that they have not actively obtained themselves. Dead lambs are rarely cached though the whole or part of those which they kill (or perhaps take as moribund lambs) may be cached. In captivity, they will temporarily cache food rather than eat it when there is something more pressing to do — such as playing with their attendant. They bolt small scraps of food as they find them but may take larger items away. The remnants of large items may be cached when hunger is satisfied. When cubs are being weaned small scraps collected by the vixen are regurgitated for them. (There is uncertainty about the behaviour of dog foxes in this respect.) Abundant sources of food, such as rubbish tips or poultry farm middens where dead birds or offal are dumped regularly, may be visited by many foxes every night. The nocturnal activities of foxes do not seem to be inhibited by bad weather. They are unafraid of water and may cross large rivers such as the middle reaches of the Wye in winter, to and fro nightly. I have no experience of the movements of foxes in the vicinity of motorways but I suspect that these would provide a tight barrier to the free movement of resident foxes.

Prospective control methods for manipulating the numbers of foxes are as follows

1. Shooting, with shotgun, by day in areas where foxes can be flushed from cover by dogs or beaters, and by night by luring them to

within gunshot distance by vocal calls.

2. Bolting foxes from their dens with terriers. Evicted foxes can be shot, netted, or, as is practised by some, killed by strong lurchers slipped when the fox flees. Cubs can be killed in their dens by terriers or dug out.

3. Gassing. Adults and cubs can be killed by introducing a hydrogen cyanide gas generating compound into earths or dens, either by a mechanical impeller or by hand.

4. Foxes can be taken in snares set on runs in fences, hedges, forest rides, scrub, and thicket.

5. Hunting with hounds whether as foot packs or with mounted hunts is practised widely in England and Wales, but is not popular north of the central lowlands of Scotland.

6. The use of leg-hold or gin traps, once responsible for killing large numbers of foxes, is now prohibited.

7. Cage traps, cumbersome and costly, are not widely used.

8. Poisons and narcotics cannot be used legally except in a rabies context.

In the event of an outbreak of rabies in foxes, swift action would be necessary to prevent the spread of the disease through the fox population. Appropriate action should

(a) effectively produce a commanding reduction in fox numbers quickly;

(b) not involve the use of dogs;

(c) be quietly conducted and not harrass the fox population;

(d) be effective at all seasons;

(e) require the minimum of skill or experience of foxes by those involved in the field; and

(f) be applicable to a wide range of environments.

Methods of control which intercept foxes during their nocturnal activities would in general be more expedient, especially over large areas, than methods which involve the pursuit or seeking out of individual foxes. Control over small areas, e.g. under 50 square km (20 square miles), depending on the environment, could include methods unsuitable for large areas.

With the exception of the use of poisons or narcotics none of the prospective methods of control would be suitable for use over large areas, since they fail to meet the criteria above;

Shooting: a, c

Bolting from dens: a, b, d, e, f

Snaring: a, e

Gin traps: a, e

Cage trapping: a, d, f

Hunting: a, b, c, e, f

The use of poisons meets the requirements entirely, or almost entirely, in all respects. Narcotics, though more attractive for humanitarian reasons, would be prohibitively laborious over large areas since narcotized animals would need to be sought and found.

The scavenging habits of the fox can be turned to good account for control purposes. Field trials of the acceptability of baits to foxes have shown that 4 oz (110 g) portions of rabbit or fish are readily taken when placed beneath turf (near likely travelling routes or foraging places such as field boundaries or headlands) at a density of about 8 bait stations per square km (20 per square mile). When bait is replenished daily the removal of 5 to 10 per cent of baits by the second day increases to 60 to 80 per cent by the eighth to fourteenth day. A similar rate of uptake is observed when the density of bait is quadrupled. Bait acceptance is high in all months except July and August. Foxes very frequently mark, with faeces, the place where the bait is laid. The incorporation in the bait of biological marker substances, such as tetracycline, reveals much about the proportion of the fox population that accept bait (if foxes are subsequently captured in the trial area) but much remains to be done. For example, it is not known how many foxes take more than one bait at given bait densities, whether or not those animals that did not appear to take bait were newcomers to the area, or whether they were subordinate animals prevented from taking bait by foxes dominant to them. Baits are taken by other species also, especially farm dogs, but there is little evidence that badgers are attracted (there was a poor uptake of bait laid near badger sets).

Such field investigations have promoted the development of a possible method of fox poisoning which would be the main plank of any anti-rabies control plan. It is intended that hidden bait would be laid, at densities of about 8 stations per square km in places that foxes are likely to frequent — rides, paths, headlands, and woodland edge — and would be replenished daily until the daily uptake shows signs of having reached its peak. Poisoned bait would then be laid. It is envisaged offering poison for only two days might, after the initial pre-baiting, remove a high proportion of the population — but since this has never been put to the test it may be found necessary in practice to offer poisoned bait for a longer period. Pre-baiting is desirable since it would reduce hazards to other species by shortening the period when poison is laid. Hiding the baits beneath turf would also diminish hazards to other species, especially birds. Bait size should be small enough to discourage the fox from taking the bait away to cache or eat elsewhere. The poison used should be safe to handle, be easily administered to the baits (10 000 bait stations would be needed over an area as large as 1250 square km (500 square miles) and rapidly immobilize the foxes so that they would be found near to the bait stations. In addition, a poison which degenerates chemically and becomes harmless after a few days would lessen the chances of other animals being poisoned if foxes carried the bait away without eating it. The universal applicability of the use of poisons will depend upon the success of investigations into the properties of prospectively suitable poisons.

Precise details of the logistics and techniques involved are not outlined here since these might soon be outdated by continuous modification in the light of current research into all aspects. Investigations on the scent secretion of foxes by two teams working independently in Britain may in due course yield useful attractant substances which if placed at the bait station could lure foxes to them more quickly. However, such attractants should not be too potent, otherwise (anthropomorphically) a fox attracted by a lure might have matters other than food on its mind when it detects the lure!

It is clear from experience overseas that anti-fox activity should be systemically conducted and be firmly controlled by a Government organization. Methods ancillary to poisoning would be used according to circumstances. Gassing, for example, would be useful if control were required in March to early April when many nursing vixens would be below ground with their cubs and would not be moving far at night. Also, following the poisoning phase dens would be stopped as part of the post-poisoning surveillance of the area for signs of the presence of foxes. The gassing of dens would require little extra effort but could add to the success of clearance. Gassing could be an important method of control in infected zones of small areas where surface cover is scarce and there is evidence of occupancy of dens.

All the foregoing considerations relate to a situation where wildlife rabies outbreaks are tightly localized. Widespread outbreaks such as occur on the Continent would need different approaches, but these will not be considered here since it involves many imponderable features.

The use of oral vaccination as a means of preventing spread of rabies is not contemplated for use in Britain. The modified live virus vaccines — used with some success experimentally in North America and Europe — may present unacceptable hazards in rabies-free areas since the vaccines currently being investigated are pathogenic to some small rodents. Thus, though foxes may be successfully vaccinated in the field, the virus might be introduced permanently into other mammalian groups.

The use of anti-fertility agents as a means of depressing the reproductive productivity of foxes and, consequently, the size of the population would involve the use of baits. Such procedures would be excessively costly (if attempted over the whole of Britain) and possibly could not be done successfully, since stringent precautions to minimize hazards to non-target species would be required. Public awareness of the large numbers of foxes in Britain (about a hundred thousand are killed annually) and the role foxes could play in a rabies outbreak has prompted many to propose a severe reduction in their numbers to a level below that required to support a wildlife outbreak. If rabies were inevitable among domestic animals and the risk of short duration this proposal would have substance — but rabies is neither inevitable nor is the risk of introduction only a passing phase. In 15 years the disease may have spread throughout France and is likely to persist — if Eastern European experience is any guide — for a long period thereafter. The expense of depressing fox numbers nationally would be enormous and the results could not be guaranteed. In addition to the unwarranted economic, ecological, and social effects of such a measure there is no justification for the slaughter of a wild animal on such a scale as a precautionary measure, against an event which is only remotely and locally probable. There is a better case for reducing the numbers of ownerless stray cats and dogs, and for imposing some restraint to the wanderings of dogs let out for the day while their owners are at work.

7

Rabies vaccines and immunity to rabies

G. S. TURNER

In the last two decades of the nineteenth century Louis Pasteur directed his attention to the study of what were then described as virus diseases. In many cases the nature of the infecting agent was unknown but smallpox was regarded as typical of such infections and remarkable because recovery from one attack left the subject lastingly immune to further attacks.

This fact and Jenner's work with vaccination against smallpox impressed Pasteur who believed that similar processes might apply to other infections. Much effort was concentrated on the possible prevention of disease by inoculation with less virulent forms of the infective agents. Pasteur's first successes were with fowl cholera and anthrax, where, after culture for several generations in an artificial medium of broth, the organisms lost their ability to produce disease. Inoculation of animals with these enfeebled organisms, however, protected them against subsequent infection with fully virulent material. This enfeeblement or attenuation was also established with rabies virus. After successive transfers in the brains of rabbits, wild or 'street' virus from the saliva of rabid animals changed its character. The long incubation time of approximately a month in the natural infection became shortened to a fixed period of 5 to 8 days. This so-called 'fixed' virus failed to infect animals unless injected directly into the brain. When inoculated by other routes, it protected animals against infection with virulent 'street' virus.

Pasteur's attenuated or 'fixed' rabies virus has been maintained in Paris and throughout the world for almost a century; it provided material for the first rabies vaccine and is still used as starting material or 'seed virus' for most of the rabies vaccines prepared today. It should also be noted that these classical researches by Pasteur and his co-workers established a model in practical immunology that has been exploited for preparing vaccines to control many other infectious diseases.

Rabies vaccines and immunity

Vaccine prepared from nervous tissue

The original rabies vaccines were suspensions of infected rabbit spinal cord that had been dried over caustic potash for different periods of time; those dried for approximately two weeks were usually non-infective, whereas those dried for shorter periods contained correspondingly more live virus. Resistance was established in dogs by the daily inoculation of cords dried for successively shorter periods. Medical history was made in July 1885 when the same technique was applied to Joseph Meister, a nine-year-old boy, who had been badly bitten by a rabid dog. Joseph did not develop the disease and furthermore survived the treatment!

The year following the introduction of rabies vaccination, some 2500 people were treated; world figures indicate that at present approximately 1·5 million people are treated annually, most of them with vaccines that differ little from those prepared almost a century ago. Certainly the Pasteur technique continued to be used in Paris until the 1950s, with all the associated problems of maintaining supplies of freshly infected rabbit cords, although these difficulties were partly resolved by storing cords in glycerine in which only minor losses of infectivity occurred. However such difficulties, and possibly a reluctance to administer large quantities of even attenuated live rabies virus to man, led workers in different parts of the world to modify Pasteur's vaccine.

Dilution of infective cords rather than desiccation was favoured by some; but most workers began to heat or chemically treat suspensions of infected nervous tissue, usually the whole brain rather than spinal cord, so that the virus was either partially or completely killed. The most notable contributor to this approach was Semple, an Englishman working in India. In 1911 he prepared vaccine in which the virus was killed by incubating infected brain suspensions with carbolic acid. The bulk of the current world production of rabies vaccine is prepared by Semple's method and it was, and probably still is, the most widely used of all the rabies vaccines.

The infected neural tissues of adult animals have provided abundant sources of virus for the production of rabies vaccines for almost a century and these notoriously crude preparations have presented the only possibility of preventing rabies infection from becoming a fatal disease. The amount of inactivated virus that they contain is several million times less than their content of brain tissue.

Reactions to nervous tissue vaccines

During the long course of injections, extending over fourteen to twenty-one days, subjects may receive up to 2·5g of brain tissue. It is this that is responsible for the severe reactions which occur in a proportion of those vaccinated. Reactions usually occur after several doses of vaccine have been administered and range from mild tingling of the hands or feet to transient paralysis. Permanent damage to the nervous system sometimes occurs and more rarely reactions are fatal. These vaccine-induced reactions have been recognized since the Pasteur era and have constantly posed a dilemma for the physician who must weigh the risk of vaccine reactions against the risk of rabies.

The substance in animal brain tissue responsible for inducing the neurological accidents described above has been identified as a protein associated with myelin — the fatty insulating material that surrounds nerves. Numerous workers have tried to prepare safer vaccines by removing this unwanted component. Rabies virus, however, binds tightly to brain tissue and these attempts have not been overwhelmingly successful. Many have resulted in substantial losses of virus and in general they have been unrewarding and uneconomic.

Myelin is absent from the nervous system of newborn animals; the brains of suckling rabbits, rats, and mice have accordingly been vigorously exploited as sources of virus for vaccine. Highly effective vaccines were first prepared from suckling mouse brain in South America in the 1950s. They have been used extensively in that area and a similar preparation is currently favoured by the Pasteur Institute in Paris. Rabies virus grows vigorously in the brains of immature animals and vaccines prepared from them are usually highly potent and can be used in reduced dosage. However surveys of the several million people vaccinated in Latin America during the last eleven years reveal that neurological accidents also occur when suckling mouse brain vaccine is administered. The likelihood of these neurological accidents occuring is four times less than that found with vaccine prepared from adult brain, but when reactions do occur with suckling mouse brain vaccine, they are more severe and more likely to be fatal.

Vaccine from avian embryos

Vaccines prepared from virus grown in non-neural tissue have obvious advantages, because of the absence of myelin, and the adaptation of several strains of rabies virus to growth in avian embryos was recorded twenty to thirty years ago. Two vaccines containing live virus grown in chick embryos have been widely and successfully used for immunizing dogs, cats, and cattle but gave disappointing results when tested in man. Vaccines containing live rabies virus are no longer recommended for human use and the administration of these vaccines is limited to animals.

During the same period, however, an inactivated vaccine suitable for human use was developed from virus grown in duck embryos. It became commercially available in the United States in 1957 and its virtual freedom from those factors known to cause neurological accidents led to its adoption as a much safer vaccine. Duck embryo vaccine has largely replaced nervous tissue vaccine in the United States where approximately 30 000 people receive antirabies treatment annually. This vaccine is also recommended for use in the United Kingdom. Retrospective studies of 420 000 subjects who received duck embryo vaccine confirmed its freedom from neurological side effects but showed that it caused very frequent local reactions. Some subjects, hypersensitive to egg protein, had severe allergic reactions.

Duck embryo vaccine has been extensively used for the immunization of those at high risk of exposure to rabies. Although most observers agree that duck embro vaccine is safer than nervous tissue vaccines, its potency has frequently been described as 'marginal', 'uncertain', or 'inconsistent'. These epithets are probably true but there is much conflicting information and no unanimity of opinion concerning the efficacy of duck embryo vaccine.

Vaccines from cultured cells

Techniques for the propagation of mammalian cells in artificial culture are by no means new. The development and exploitation of such cell cultures for the growth of viruses received much impetus from Enders and his co-workers in 1949. They grew polio virus in cultures of monkey kidney cells from which a very efficient polio vaccine was subsequently prepared.

A further decade elapsed, however, before rabies virus was successfully propagated in cultures of non-neural cells. A great many cell systems were subsequently investigated as substrates for the growth of the virus and although many cell types supported its growth, the highest yields of virus were only obtained in cultures unacceptable for use in man. Several highly successful veterinary vaccines were developed in these cells but progress with cell-culture vaccines for human use was disappointingly slow.

The governments of most countries have committees and departments which examine new medicines and immunological products. These licensing authorities rightly have exacting requirements for the cell substrates used for human vaccine production. They usually permit the use of primary cultures, i.e. cells cultivated for the first time from the tissues of selected stocks of animals; if human cells are used, cultures must be of known origin and the cells must possess the normal diploid (double set) of chromosomes. All cells must of course be free from extraneous viruses. It is also recommended that rabies virus in vaccines for human use should be inactivated. Adequate potency in inactivated vaccines usually requires a high initial virus content. This imposes a further restriction since adequate virus yields are difficult to achieve in these cell systems.

Despite these difficulties several vaccines of cell-culture origin have been developed for use in man, and are either already licensed or in clinical trial. The earliest of these was prepared in primary hamster kidney cells in Canada in 1960 and a vaccine prepared in similar cells was extensively tested in man in the Soviet Union. The safety and potency of both these preparations is satisfactorily established and licences have been granted for their use in their countries of origin. In Western Europe and the United States, however, they have not had wide acceptance and attention is currently directed towards a vaccine prepared in cultures of human cells. These cells, designated as human diploid cell strain (HDCS) or Wistar Institute (WI38) cells, fulfil the requirements described above and have already been accepted as substrates for other virus vaccines.

Initial trials of HDCS vaccine in monkeys showed that a single dose gave far superior immune responses (i.e. more specific resistance) than did similar doses of brain tissue or duck embryo vaccine and that the animals were protected against subsequent experimental infection with wild strains of rabies virus. More important, it was demonstrated that a single dose given several hours *after* experimental infection protected more monkeys than did fourteen daily doses of duck embryo vaccine. HDCS vaccine has now had extensive trials in many thousands of human volunteers in the United States, the Middle East, and Europe including the United Kingdom, where long-term studies are now in their third year. The reports of these many trials are unanimous. All record a striking immune response in those vaccinated and all draw attention to the absence of other than minor local reactions. The difficulties that hindered the large-scale production of the vaccine appear to have been resolved. Nevertheless not all workers are convinced that human diploid cells are ideal for the production of rabies vaccines; certainly their control and the necessity to concentrate virus harvests make the vaccine costly to prepare, and the search for other suitable cell substrates continues.

Vaccines and vaccination for animals

The vaccination of domestic animals — particularly cats and dogs — has been outstandingly successful in the control of rabies. In countries where the disease is endemic in wildlife, or where for geographical reasons quarantine is impracticable, adequate canine immunization is a major factor in preventing the spread of the disease to man. Properly administered, the currently used veterinary vaccines will immunize 90 per cent to 100 per cent of dogs and cats. Coverage of not less than 70 per cent of the canine population is sufficient to break the chain of transmission among them and extinguish the disease.

A Semple-type vaccine was first used in 1921 for the successful mass vaccination of dogs in Japan. Subsequently, controlled studies were conducted in different parts of the world. Various types of vaccine containing either live-attenuated or killed virus have been tested, and their efficiency and the duration of the immunity they confer is well established. In general longer lasting immunity is obtained with the veterinary vaccines containing live virus and the necessity for revaccination is less frequent. However, these products require careful storage at low temperatures, since their immunizing power depends upon their content of live virus. Furthermore, the live virus in some types is still virulent for young puppies, cattle, cats, and some exotic animals. Nevertheless these vaccines have been highly successful in rabies eradication campaigns throughout the world and for this purpose compare favourably with more recent vaccines prepared in tissue cultures. Many workers, however, question the wisdom of using live virus vaccines even for animals and there are now many potent inactivated veterinary vaccines available.

Apart from the immediate hazards to man posed by canine rabies, the disease is also the source of grave economic losses to the cattle industry in several parts of the world. Mexico and Latin America are most affected but the fox-borne epizooty is responsible for many bovine infections in Europe as well. Extensive laboratory and field evaluation has proved that suitable vaccination programmes mainly using modified live virus preparations can effectively reduce these losses.

Vaccination of wild life
Population reduction has so far failed to solve the problem of wildlife rabies, and gassing, shooting, and poisoning are unpopular with wildlife conservationists. The application of vaccination to control rabies in wild animals, particularly foxes, is receiving serious attention in North America and Europe at the present time. Attenuated live virus, given by mouth, has been shown to induce an immune response in foxes. A variety of methods of administering vaccine by this route is being examined. Prepared baits are being sought which are acceptable to foxes and in which the virus is stable. The virulence for other species of the live virus in the vaccine is also being carefully examined, and the investigators believe that all these problems can be solved.

Dosage and administration of vaccines
It has already been mentioned that the traditional vaccines prepared from neural tissues contain only very small amounts of rabies virus or 'antigen'. This paucity of antigen was believed to necessitate a prolonged series of daily injections extending over two or three weeks. Modern immunological practice does not support this belief, but in the face of an invariably fatal disease it is perhaps understandable that

these heroic measures persist. It may also be pertinent to dispel another misconception: rabies vaccines are commonly inoculated beneath the skin of the abdomen − *not* into the stomach or abdominal cavity − because of the large area available in all but the leanest subjects. Sites for fourteen to twenty-one doses in the arms become difficult to find and multiple doses in the buttocks are painful to sit on!

In many countries, however, modern vaccines are successfully administered in much abbreviated courses, four to six doses being sufficient to induce very rapid immune responses. It has also been shown recently that very small doses of potent cell-culture vaccine, inoculated into, not under, the skin, may be as effective as much larger doses given into the muscles.

Two major applications of rabies vaccination should be distinguished. First, the control of rabies in animals and the immunization of persons at risk *before* they are exposed to the disease is widely practised. Countless laboratory experiments and field trials have shown that this is highly effective in protecting animals and there are no records of human rabies occurring in individuals known to be immune at the time of exposure. Secondly there is active immunization *after* possible infection. Pasteurian in origin, this practice is considered to be reasonable because the time of infection by animal bite can usually be determined precisely, and the incubation time of the natural disease is usually prolonged. This long incubation period theoretically allows time for immune responses to vaccine to occur before the onset of the disease.

It is difficult to prove the value of this 'post-exposure' vaccination. Many subjects receiving treatment may not be infected, for, despite popular mythology, man is relatively resistant to rabies and natural infection is therefore uncertain. It is, of course, ethically impossible to withold treatment, and so controlled studies cannot be made. Until recently no animal models, including Pasteur's original experiments, convincingly demonstrated a protective effect of vaccine administered *after* infection. The retrospective examination of more than a million cases of post-exposure treatment in the 1940s also permitted no conclusions to be drawn. The most credible evidence of its value in man comes from a twenty-year survey in India where 56 per cent of untreated exposed subjects died of rabies whereas only 7 per cent died after treatment.

The results of recent animal experiments with highly potent cell-culture vaccines have been more encouraging. Significant reductions in mortality were demonstrated in mice and monkeys treated with single doses of these preparations *after* experimental infection. It seems likely therefore that despite the reservations of some workers concerning the value of post-exposure vaccine treatment, the recent cell-culture vaccines will prove far safer and provide much greater possibilities of protection than those used hitherto.

Vaccines and immunity

The body has more than one way of expressing specific protective immunity to infection and in responding to vaccination. One of these is the production of soluble substances associated with the serum proteins of the blood. These are usually described as 'circulating' or 'humoral' antibodies. The other response is associated directly with cellular activity and known as 'cell-mediated' immunity. The respective roles of these two aspects of the immune response to rabies are still under investigation; certainly cell-mediated effects are imperfectly understood.

Antirabies serum

Much more is known about the antibodies that neutralize rabies virus. Serum antibody in animals and man can be estimated with reasonable accuracy and the amount present is used to assess immune responses. In experimental animals, many workers have demonstrated a correlation between the amount of antibody present in the blood and resistance to subsequent infection. In individuals who are already infected, the role of antibody induced by the classic method of vaccine treatment is difficult to explain. Antibody is not usually detectable until seven or more days after starting vaccination in animals and man. Vaccination is therefore unlikely to be effective in severe infections where the incubation period may be short. Many individuals dying of rabies have massive amount of neutralizing antibody late in their infection, suggesting that antibody appearing at this time does not affect the lethal outcome of the disease. Some workers believe that antibody alone may only prolong the time to death and that some antibody components are actually involved in the disease process or 'pathogenesis' of rabies. Most evidence suggests that once the infection has reached the central nervous system, antibody is ineffective. However, many animal experiments have demonstrated that antibody protects if it is administered before virus has reached the central nervous system. The administration of antirabies serum, as well as vaccine, within twenty-four to forty-eight hours of infection is recommended practice in all severe exposures to rabies.

The most convincing evidence of the value of antirabies serum in man was demonstrated twenty years ago. This unique and dramatic incident occurred in an Iranian village where a rabid wolf bit twenty-nine people in succession. All twenty-nine were transported to Teheran where they received an intensive course of vaccination. Seventeen also received one or two injections of anti-rabies serum; only one of these died compared with three of the remaining twelve who received only vaccine. The figures are even more dramatic if only those with severe head wounds are considered; 75 per cent of those who had only vaccine died compared with 14 per cent of those receiving serum and vaccine.

The administration of antirabies serum is not without hazard. Antirabies serum is prepared in animals and the inoculation of animal sera into man often causes severe reactions or 'serum sickness'. This problem is likely to decrease, however, for the exceptional amounts of antibody recently obtained in man with cell-culture vaccines are making it possible to acquire a stock of human antirabies serum from blood donated by immunized volunteers. Because this material is of human origin it does not cause unwelcome reactions in human recipients.

The combined use of antiserum and vaccine is complicated by the fact that responses to vaccine are partially suppressed by antibody. The amounts and spacing of the doses of both antirabies serum and vaccine must be carefully adjusted if the effects of one are not to cancel out the effects of the other.

Rabies vaccines and interferon

It was observed, approximately twenty years ago, that the growth of one virus in a host cell prevented the growth of a second virus. This viral interference was found to be due to the release of a soluble material by the cell which was named 'interferon'. Interferon activity is species-specific, that is mouse interferon acts only on the growth of virus in mouse cells, rabbit interferon on its growth in rabbit cells and so on. The reaction is not an immunological one, and is not specific against any particular virus; indeed, interferon will prevent the growth of a wide variety of viruses both in cultured cells and in intact animals.

It was subsequently found that interferon could be induced by a number of synthetic non-virus materials. Recent animal experiments showed that if interferon was induced by viruses or synthetic inducers at or around the time of infection, several species of laboratory animals could be protected against rabies. Interferon induction may be one mechanism by which rabies vaccines afford protection, for although interferon induction is not usually exhibited by traditional vaccines, several highly concentrated cell-culture vaccines that protected animals in single doses induced interferon before antibody appeared. It seems possible therefore that interferon may also be exploited as part of the arsenal for the treatment of rabies.

Future vaccines

It was predicted almost ten years ago that future rabies vaccines might contain only those components of the virus that were active in inducing immunity. These 'subunits' of the virus would contain no genetic material either from the virus or from the host in which it was grown; and tests of some early 'subunit' vaccines showed that they induced substantial immune responses in man and animals.

The cultivation of rabies virus in cell cultures has facilitated purification and given impetus to the systematic investigation of the chemical, physical, and biological properties of the virus particle. Several structures associated with particular functions were identified when the purified virus was disrupted. It is now known, for example, that the material which induces antibody responses and protects animals is associated with the spikes seen on the surface of the virus (see Chapter 2). The chemical composition of this material has already been determined and the methods for its experimental isolation established. If it could be produced economically it is possible that even safer and more active vaccines might be prepared.

Index

Index

Index